Amrit Yoga &
the Yoga Sutras

Other Books by Yogi Amrit Desai
Kripalu Yoga: Meditation in Motion, Books I and II
Working Miracles of Love
Happiness is Now
Amrit Yoga: Explore, Expand and
Experience the Spiritual Depth of Yoga
Upcoming: Love & Bliss

Amrit Yoga &
the Yoga Sutras

Amrit Yoga and Its Roots in
Patanjali's Ashtanga Yoga

by
Yogi Amrit Desai

Red Elixir | Rhinebeck, NY   Yoga Network International | Salt Springs, FL

Published by Yoga Network International, Inc.
PO Box 5340
Salt Springs, FL 32134
www.amritkala.com

in co-operation with
Red Elixir
27 Lamoree Road
Rhinebeck, NY 12572

Cover design by J. Rogers Design, St. Petersburg, FL
Book design by T. Cruse Design, Philadelphia, PA
Teaching photographs by Peter Goldberg
Back and inside cover portraits by Heather Titus
Painting of Dadaji courtesy of the Kayavarohan Temple
ISBN 0-9719455-0-0

Table of Contents

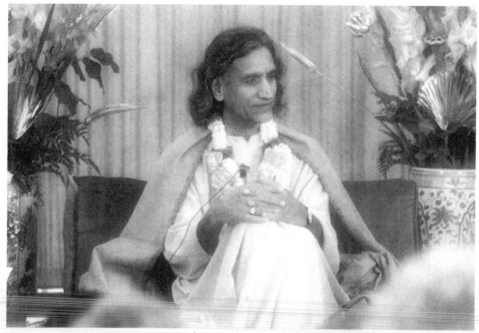

Introduction

Nothing compares with the direct experience of being in the presence of a great spiritual teacher. There is no substitute for the depth of transformation that can occur for the student who is open and receptive to the wisdom only a true master can impart. Yogi Amrit Desai, known as Gurudev, is one such rare being. He possesses the unique ability to transmit the esoteric scriptural truths of the ages in a profound experiential way that we can all apply to truly transform our lives. Passed down from teacher to student for centuries, usually via the oral tradition, these sacred truths are the very kernel of the essence of life—they provide us with the means to discover what we all seek.

That said, I have nevertheless made a sincere attempt to bring the treasure trove of Yogi Desai's teachings to the written page. I have faithfully adhered to his sometimes circular style of speaking and writing to maintain the richness of his language. I encourage the reader to feel these teachings rather than try to understand them on a mental level. This is as close as you can come to receiving the depth of these teachings through the medium of the written word. Yogi Desai's teachings are so vast and all-encompassing, it would be difficult to contain it all in a single book. Therefore, this volume is dedicated to the authentic basis of his teachings in the exposition known as the Yoga Sutras. Its author, Yogi Patanjali, is a vague figure who lived some 2,000 years ago. Little is known about him, except for his invaluable contribution to the study of yoga. Prior to Patanjali, yogic principles were held in secret by a privileged few. For the first time, he codified these precious truths into simple yet mysterious statements that confound students to this day.

In the following pages, Yogi Desai's brilliant perspective on the hidden meanings behind Patanjali's mystical phrases are revealed. Absorb them, savor them and discover how pertinent and applicable they are to life today, using the experiential techniques of Amrit Yoga. The writings in this book are the perpetual inspiration of Yogi Desai, but it has come to fruition due to the painstaking diligence of many devotees. I would like to gratefully acknowledge those whose hands, hearts and dedication have contributed to preparing this work: Kamini Desai and Megan Wardrop, associate editors; Malay Desai and Urmila Desai, for their unswerving devotion and selfless service; Karen Bhakti Platt, James Amarish Caruso and Donna Surekha Ireland, senior Amrit Yoga teachers; Marian Yashodhara Betty, Patricia Vrajdipa Stevens, Doug Sanjay Martin and Federico Giller, fellow travelers on this path.

Lila Ivey, Editor
(Modini)
Sumneytown, PA
February 2002

ॐ

1

Yoga for the 21st Century

The term "yoga" means union or oneness. It describes a state of unity consciousness that is infinite, whole, ever new and fresh—a state of being that is untouched by time, cultural conditioning, or religious doctrine. The ancient rishis, seers who had a direct experience of God through yogic practices, realized this great truth thousands of years ago. It wasn't until Yogi Patanjali codified these secret truths that the sacred science of yoga became known. Patanjali provided others with a method to connect with the inner source of life itself.

Yoga has not changed in the past six thousand years, but what we call yoga has changed significantly. As the teachings traveled through time, they collected the dust of human unconsciousness. Eventually, that which lingered in society was merely the form of yoga while much of the spirit was lost. We have been left with a *philosophy* of oneness rather than an *experience* of oneness.

Fortunately, there have always been a few great yogis who renewed and revitalized yoga through the centuries, making it available to the world. In 1893, Swami Vivekananda was the first to introduce yoga to the West. Others followed, Paramahansa Yogananda in 1920, then Maharishi Mahesh Yogi and Swami Muktananda in the 1960s. In their own way, they each taught about the unity and connected sacredness of life, which is the foundation of yoga.

For many years, however, there were no masters teaching the true, in-depth practice of Hatha Yoga in the West. The teaching of postures as a physical discipline became very popular. But postures are only the tip of the iceberg—the outermost part of yoga. The subtler, more internal aspects are invisible and are often missed in the current practice of Hatha Yoga.

Still, these yoga practices met the needs of many: holistic health practitioners, athletes, dancers, therapists and businessmen. Yoga programs were developed by stress clinics, health resorts, gymnasiums, spas, diet clinics, and drug rehab centers. As uninformed teachers capitalized on the growing acceptance of yoga, it grew in breadth but not depth. Such popularized versions in some ways undermined and compromised the original intent of yoga.

As yoga continued to be westernized, numerous books were published that focused exclusively on its therapeutic applications. This is not to say those innovative practices were incorrect. On the contrary, the widespread popularity of yoga proves that they had a profound impact. The worldwide adoption of yoga is proof that even the popular versions of yoga did fulfill many needs of society. Now, however, the time has come to recapture the original spirit of yoga without sacrificing the wide range of applications present today.

It is time to explore yoga's depth in addition to its breadth. The need is emerging throughout our culture. Those from every walk of life are waking up to a deep spiritual hunger. The abundance of new books and magazine articles reveal this craving for deeper values.

Understood correctly, Hatha Yoga is capable of using the body and the mind to transcend the limits ordinarily imposed by both body and mind. That is also the basis of Amrit Yoga. It is a non-aggressive, non-competitive, nonmental response to the primal wisdom of prana—our evolutionary life force. Ultimately, the practice leads to union of the individual soul with the infinite cosmic soul. And that is the real purpose of yoga.

I invite us all to embrace a renewed vision of yoga's potential. The time is ripe to move into its deeper, unexplored dimensions. Yoga is a complete approach to integrating body, mind and spirit, and that integration is what brings us into unity consciousness. More than ever, the world needs to reconnect with its innate wholeness and divinity. Yoga has both the breadth and the depth to lead the way.

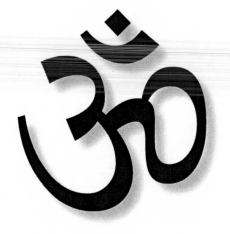

II
Traditional Paths of Yoga

All systems of yoga seek the same final goal–liberation or enlightenment. The various branches may be different entryways, but they arrive at the same destination. Actually, you cannot practice just one branch of yoga exclusively without the other branches of yoga being part of it in the process. For example, you cannot practice Karma Yoga, the yoga of selfless service, without bringing in the Bhakti Yoga of love and devotion. One will remain incomplete without the other. Love and meditative awareness are the two powerful integrative principles that are at the core of all disciplines of yoga. The major branches include:

Patanjali's Aahtanga (Eight-Limbed) Yoga
Hatha And Raja Yoga

When Yogi Patanjali (circa 200 BC) called his exposition of yoga Ashtanga, he chose this word consciously to describe the eight limbs that are the extensions of the one body of yoga. If he had chosen eight steps of yoga, it would have made yoga a linear practice, one step at a time, like going up a ladder. However, just as all the limbs of the human body function in co-creation for any physical expression, similarly, all limbs of the body of Ashtanga Yoga must function harmoniously for the fulfillment of the purpose of yoga, which is union. Yoga practice that does not integrate the entire body of yoga remains incomplete. When you work with each limb individually you divide the core of yoga. When any one limb is exclusively isolated from the others, it fails to create integration among the conflicting aspects of our being.

This means that the eight-limbed body of Ashtanga Yoga forms a holistic system. Hatha Yoga can be practiced with a primary focus on the external form as a foundation for the spiritual dimensions of the whole body of Ashtanga Yoga. Even when the physical discipline is practiced alone, it can be impregnated with intention to plant the seeds of the mental and spiritual dimensions that expand Hatha Yoga from an exclusively physical discipline into a psychosomatic and bio-spiritual discipline.

Wherever you go, whatever you do, all the limbs of your body function and act in co-creation. Can you enter a room with just one part of your body? Of course not. So just as you cannot walk into a room with only one part of your body, you cannot fulfill the true purpose of the practice of yoga unless you integrate the whole body of Ashtanga Yoga, regardless of which particular limb is predominantly active. When you engage the whole body of yoga you maximize the power of yoga.

Our being represents the integrated expression of all of our bodies: physical body, prana body, mental body, intellectual body, and the bliss body. When every level of our being manifests into active expression, it is the experience of yoga.

Our physical body is the external part of our being; the mind and heart are the internal parts of our being and the soul is the source of life of the body, mind, heart and spirit. When we fully enter our being, it is the harmonious interactive co-creation of the body, mind, heart and soul.

The body alone cannot enter the sacred sanctuary of being. It must be integrated and whole. That is yoga.

Ashtanga Yoga is composed of the yamas and niyamas, asanas, pranayama, pratyahara, dharana, dhyana and samadhi. The yamas and niyamas are the observances and disciplines that protect you from internal and external disturbances and assure the successful practice of Ashtanga Yoga.

Asanas and pranayama represent the discipline of the body (Hatha Yoga). Pratyahara and dharana represent the discipline of the mind; dhyana turns the entire practice of Ashtanga Yoga into a spiritual discipline (Raja Yoga). Dhyana is the only part of Ashtanga Yoga that has the power and the potential to create dynamic integration where the body, mind, heart and soul can function as a harmonious whole. The moment you remove the meditative aspect of the practice, it is impossible to fulfill the intention of the practice of yoga, which is integration of all aspects of our being.

You can divide Ashtanga Yoga into external and internal. In Amrit Yoga, you begin with the external form of asana and pranayama as an entry point to develop the spiritual dimension that transcends the form into formlessness. The practice of yoga leads to transcendence of the limitations of both the body and the mind and into the experience of samadhi where all aspects of our being melt into the integrated experience of yoga.

Hatha Yoga: The Yoga Of Physical Discipline

In Amrit Yoga, asanas and pranayama are performed as a preparation. They establish the foundation for the mental and spiritual dimension of Raja Yoga, which includes pratyahara, dharana and dhyana. Even though Hatha Yoga appears to be a physical discipline, it invariably carries within it the components of Raja Yoga. It is a journey from external to internal; from form to formlessness; from physical to spiritual.

7

Raja Yoga: Classical Or Royal Yoga

The successful foundation of Raja Yoga is built on internal focus and meditative awareness during the practice of asana and pranayama. You cannot perform any physical act without the mind being part of it; neither can you perform any mental act without the body being an integral part. The body-mind is in co-creation in every action. Devoid of the mental and spiritual components, the discipline of Hatha Yoga remains incomplete.

Bhakti Yoga: The Yoga Of Devotion

The way of transcendent love sees the whole universe, animate and inanimate, as being pervaded by divinity. On this heart-centered path, devotees believe in a Supreme Being that is not separate from the material world and perceive the presence of the Creator in His creation. They embrace all of creation with unconditional love. Practitioners perform ritual offerings such as flowers, incense, chanting and meditating on the Supreme Being with whom they feel moved to connect. They use the chanting of mantras, music and dance as integral parts of their practice to express their devotion and love for God. The devotees of Bhakti Yoga predominantly follow the path of love and devotion to merge with the divine.

Jnana Yoga: The Yoga Of Wisdom

The Jnana yogi finds God through knowledge. It teaches the ideal of non-dualism—that reality is singular and your perception of countless distinct phenomena is a basic misconception. At enlightenment, everything melts into one, and you become one with the divine, immortal spirit. Jnana Yoga is the yoga of the philosopher and thinker who wants to go beyond the visible, material reality. This is the path of the yogi who wishes to realize the underlying unity behind diversity predominantly through the path of intellect.

Karma Yoga: The Yoga Of Selfless Service

Karma yogis remove the separation of the ego-self from the all pervading Self by performing selfless service to humanity and all living beings. This is their way of transcending their separative egos and achieving union with God through right action. This path's most important principle is to act unselfishly and perform service for its own sake, without attachment, and with integrity. Practitioners believe that our actions, whether bodily, vocal or mental, have far-reaching consequences (karma) for which we must assume full responsibility. By letting go of the self-image in the service of the Self that is the Self of all, karma yogis experience union with the higher Self.

Mantra Yoga: The Yoga Of Sound

Mantras are sacred sounds of power. When they are practiced with love, faith, dedication, meditative attention and absorption, they become vehicles of transformation of body, mind, heart and soul. Each mantra corresponds with a specific force and holds within it a magical potency that can be released through the continuous, one-pointed, meditative absorption in the practice of mantra. This power of mantra is unlocked through repetition that purifies all of the bodies– physical, mental and emotional–transforming consciousness. Traditionally, practitioners receive a mantra from a guru during a formal initiation.

Tantra Yoga: The Yoga Of Surrender

Tantra is the most complex and most widely misunderstood branch. In the West and in India, Tantra is often confused with spiritualized sex. While sexual rituals are used in some schools of Tantra, this isn't a regular practice in the majority of schools. Tantra is actually a strict spiritual discipline involving complex rituals and detailed visualizations of deities. Tantra enlists Shakti, the feminine principle of cosmic existence, in the quest for the divine. Adepts affirm that the body is the temple of the divine and is an invaluable instrument for reaching liberation. Tantra accepts the reality of all that is present in life with mindful awareness.

Another name for Tantra is Kundalini Yoga, which literally means "She who is coiled." It hints at the secret serpent power that Tantra seeks to activate, a latent spiritual energy stored in the human body that lies dormant at the base of the spine. True Kundalini Yoga is total surrender to God. Absolute surrender is the very core of the practice of Kundalini Yoga.

III

What is Amrit Yoga?

A mrit Yoga connects yoga practice with the ancient roots and fundamental principles as codified by Patanjali that are at the core of all branches of yoga. By adding the mental and spiritual disciplines of Raja Yoga, inwardly focused attention and meditative awareness, Amrit Yoga combines the strengths of Hatha and Raja Yoga into one system.

The entire system of Amrit Yoga is intended to lead practitioners to move toward the awakening of Shakti and the higher integrative centers of consciousness. The core of Hatha Yoga practice is willful; the core of Kundalini Yoga practice is surrender. Amrit Yoga is the outcome of prana awakening, the stage prior to the awakening of Kundalini. It is designed to develop willful practice toward surrender of our self-image and self-concepts that keep us from connecting to the Source of our being.

Amrit Yoga can be a powerful extension for yoga teachers and students from all traditions who wish to add the spiritual dimension into their personal practice and professional skills. It uses the body as an entry point to explore, experience and release psychosomatic blocks that prevent us from tapping into the source of the infinite potential within. It creates new possibilities for widening the range of healing modalities and Self-discovery.

The practice of Amrit Yoga cultivates inward focus and meditative awareness along with postures and pranayamas. Inward focus becomes an anchor for engaging scattered attention. Withdrawing attention from internal and external disturbances (pratyahara) and focusing on bodily sensations (dharana) heals the body-mind split, bringing the mind and body into a harmonious, co-creative friendship. Internal focus is the single most powerful tool in preventing chronic unconscious, unproductive mental dialogues, images and emotional reactions. Unconscious habits accompany us through every activity all day long; the yoga mat is not an exception.

The vigorous traditions of Hatha Yoga provide powerful physical results and are intended to serve as a foundation for the mental and spiritual dimensions of yoga. Hard work can silence the mind during vigorous practice, but has no power to transcend or alter emotional and karmic patterns held securely in the unconscious. Vigorous practice combined with internal focus engages the mental and emotional bodies in the practice of yoga—expanding its scope and deepening the experience of Hatha Yoga many fold. For your body to be the temple of the divine, your yoga practice must harness and harmonize the conflicting forces and disturbances that arise from the body, emotions and mind. These unconscious forces keep you divided and fragmented in your thinking, feeling and doing.

Amrit Yoga is a metaphor for life. The skills of mindful attention and meditative awareness you develop on the yoga mat extend to challenges you encounter in life. Painful transition periods, relationships and crises can become opportunities and openings for personal transformation. The practice of Amrit Yoga has the power to engage you totally, absorb you completely, and integrate you fully in body, mind, heart and soul. It empowers you to enter the experience of unity and ecstasy, which is integral to the experience of yoga.

The Purpose Of Yoga

The purpose for the practice of yoga is to enter the integrated state of our being. The body is used as a vehicle through which we recognize the blockages that keep us from our being. They exist not only on the physical but also on the mental and emotional levels. Yoga postures are used as a vehicle to bring these blockages to the surface to be reintegrated.

The first stage of Amrit Yoga is willful practice where we learn to face our psychosomatic tensions. As we go deeper to the subtler levels, we awaken the underlying layers that are accompanied by old memories, fears, shame and anger. In the practice of Amrit Yoga, you learn to encounter these blockages with meditative attention and to release them the moment you encounter them. These subtler layers of tension that live in the form of unconscious habits and preprogrammed attitudes are the cause of ongoing stress. The possibility of releasing and integrating these tensions comes from fully experiencing them without distorting them with anticipation, expectation and evaluation.

We can use yoga postures to transcend both physical as well as more subtle layers of tension and limitation. Inward focus and meditative awareness allow you to dive beneath the ordinary surface level of waking consciousness into a state of awakened consciousness that acts independently of your acquired personal limitations. As you enter this depth in the practice of Amrit Yoga, the postures simultaneously become therapeutic and spiritual in nature.

When we exclusively focus on the physical dimension of yoga, the depth of our practice cannot go beyond form to experience the formless spirit of yoga.

The basic intention in the practice of Amrit Yoga is to

consolidate and integrate the fragmentation of mental, emotional and energetic forces, bringing all parts of your being into balance.

Amrit Yoga uses Hatha Yoga postures as a foundation to bring about nadi shuddhi–the purification of the body's nerve channels, balancing the function of glands and ridding the body of toxins. This simultaneously retards the aging process and increases vitality, endurance and flexibility. To confine the profound depth of yoga and to use it exclusively as a body-centered practice is like clipping the wings of an airplane and using it is an automobile. The purpose of Amrit Yoga is to give wings to your practice to explore, expand and experience the infinite power of spirit that you are.

As you proceed into the second stage, which focuses on prolonged holding of the posture with inward focus and meditative awareness, you experience the unique blending of the physical, mental and spiritual dimensions of the practice of yoga. Meditative attention and awareness anchor all the psychosomatic forces, inducing them to function harmoniously as a unit. Yoga postures, integrated with inward focus, allow you to engage all levels of your being, helping release tensions that surface during the practice of the postures.

The limits we experience in our physical, mental and spiritual expressions are acquired and stored in our subconscious over many lifetimes (karma). Our body and our unconscious hold the entire history of what we have lived through and experienced. During the practice of Amrit Yoga, you intentionally bring to the surface these blockages built into your unconscious memories and muscles as chronic tensions. As you enter deeper and deeper levels, you begin to experience catharsis. All such past limitations, inhibitions and boundaries from living unconsciously can only be released through practicing yoga with consciousness.

Your body is not your enemy. It is not some entity to fight with in order to overcome its weaknesses.

Being in direct contact with your body without self-criticism or struggle is the first step toward being in touch with who you really are. Only when there is total acceptance of your body's strengths and weaknesses is there the possibility for you to befriend your body.

In the practice of Amrit Yoga, postures are used as a foundation for self-study, self-observation and self-discovery. The process of exploring, experiencing and entering the deeper layers reveals the truth that your self-concepts deny, cover up or fight with.

What makes the real difference in the practice of Amrit Yoga is the penetrating power of inward focus and meditative awareness. Together they work through the chronic source of tension that lives beneath the surface, helping us break through suppressed emotional memories, fears and defenses that keep us from being in direct contact with our divine Source. When you enter the deepest level of integrated being, the actor and the achiever disappear and only the action remains. When you are integrated, your energy operates in complete harmony—you become deeply absorbed, integrated and whole.

In the absence of internal conflict, there is no loss of energy.

When you are undivided and whole, your unconscious muscular, mental and energy blocks dissolve and merge into the integrated state of your being. When you move out of doing, you merge into being. When you are engaged by meditative awareness, you have the freedom to travel freely through your thinking, acting and feeling centers. Everything that you do becomes regenerative rather than depleting. In the absence of

15

internal conflict, you spontaneously enter the deepest levels of relaxation. Only when your mind is not struggling to control your body does your higher power take over. You merge into your spiritual being. When you are totally present you are able to let your body reveal its strengths and weaknesses rather than relying on pre-programmed selfconcepts that tell you what you can and cannot do.

Amrit Yoga is the ecstatic union between the primal energy of Shakti, manifesting in its purity, dancing with Shiva consciousness. The principles of Amrit Yoga that you integrate in performing yoga on the mat are not just applicable for increased efficiency in the practice of yoga, but also increased ability to encounter the obstacles and challenges that you face in your personal and professional life. What you learn in formal practice becomes a tool in the fieldwork of your daily life. Your yoga practice is not limited to the yoga mat but extends through every interaction—in your relationship with yourself, with your loved ones and with the world you live in.

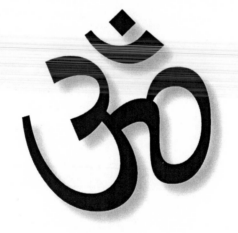

IV

The Amrit Yoga Lineage of Masters

Yogi Amrit Desai is a descendant of one of the most esoteric yogic traditions of India, the path of Shaktipat Kundalini Yoga. The teachings of Kundalini Yoga date back thousands of years, when the austere life of a yogi consisted of isolation and meditation. Arising from deep states of meditation, their postures flowed smoothly, without any conscious effort on their part. It was during such intense spiritual practice that the ancient yogis experienced what came to be known as Hatha Yoga. The postures were not learned; they emerged spontaneously. This phenomenon was the outgrowth of the awakened Kundalini Shakti, the divine energy that lies dormant within us all. This is the origin of yoga postures, pranayamas, kriyas, locks, mudras, dance and music. The entire system of yoga is not man-made, but a direct gift from God.

The unity consciousness they attained was a state of being that exists beyond the limitations of time, untouched by cultural conditioning or religious doctrine. The rishis realized the great truth they had experienced, so when they spoke of yoga, they spoke of it as a sacred science. To them, yoga meant connecting with the inner source of life itself. In ancient times, these sacred teachings were passed down to only a chosen few, from guru to disciple. Yogi Desai received these age-old secrets of yoga directly from his guru, Swami Shri Kripalvanandji, one of the greatest Kundalini masters of this century. The life of Swami Shri Kripalvanandji, lovingly known as Kripalu or Bapuji by his followers, is an amazing story of unswerving devotion.

Lila Ivey, Editor

The Path Of Kripalu

From childhood, Kripalu possessed a burning desire for communion with God. As a teenager he would chant japa (mantra repetition) throughout the night or perform puja (worship) to Lord Shiva until dawn, pouring streams of water over his statue of Shiva until the streets ran wet. Passersby on their way to work the next morning would wonder where so much water had come from in the absence of rain.

By the age of 19, Kripalu's desire for God-realization had become so intense, and his attempts to achieve it so frustrating, that in despair he had already attempted suicide three times. It was as he contemplated his fourth attempt that he met the one who would soon become his guru.

One night, he planned to throw himself in front of a train and end his suffering. Praying for the last time in his favorite temple, Kripalu cried out: "Divine Mother, why did I have to live such a worthless life? Oh Mother, permit me to merge into thy holy feet!" As he sobbed, he felt the presence of another who silently put a tender hand on his shoulder.

"My son, do not consider taking your life. Do not cry, come along, come along...," came the loving voice. Stunned, Kripalu fell into the arms of the kind stranger. He had told no one of his suicide plans. Wordlessly, he rose and followed the stranger.

The following day, Kripalu visited the ashram of the stranger, who he learned went by the name Dadaji. As he was being ushered into Dadaji's darshan room, he was greeted eagerly by the assembled disciples, many of whom were Bombay's wealthiest citizens. They had been told four months earlier that on that day would come the young man who would become Dadaji's foremost disciple.

Perplexed and embarrassed at being so suddenly thrust into the spotlight, Kripalu, who was at that time penniless and living on a few handfuls of chickpeas a day, demurred at this suggestion. Dadaji went on to assure him that he would eventually don the orange robes of the swami order and renounce the world. Kripalu protested that he was certain he was not ready to completely renounce his material desires. This was a characteristic response of Kripalu's deep humility.

At Dadaji's request, Kripalu moved into the ashram and made it his home, and thus began fifteen months of close personal training and attention that was to totally transform his life. Kripalu became Dadaji's chief disciple and spokesman, and as his contact with his guru continued, his love for his teacher filled his entire being.

Kripalu noted that many miraculous events occurred during this period of training. For example, two or three hundred disciples came to the ashram every day. Despite the large number of visitors, Dadaji knew everyone's name and even spoke to them in their native language without a visible clue as to what language they spoke.

On another occasion, Kripalu and Dadaji went for a long walk along the beach one evening during the course of which it became clear to Kripalu that although Dadaji was perfectly visible to him as they carried on their conversation, he was invisible to everyone else they encountered along the way. When they returned to the ashram, Kripalu discovered that Dadaji had also been present at the ashram giving darshan the entire time. He was in awe to discover that Dadaji had the ability to be in two places at once.

Many times, Kripalu experienced the wonders of Dadaji's miraculous inner powers, but Kripalu's natural skepticism always kept him from accepting some of the yogic powers he witnessed. Once when Kripalu questioned him about his age, Dadaji avoided answering, but Kripalu persisted and finally Dadaji replied: "I am a year and 3/4 old," but this only confused Kripalu more. Dadaji told him, "This is a mystery to be revealed to you in the future." With this, Kripalu's imagination soared, so Dadaji consoled him by saying that only at the proper time would Kripalu come to know his true identity.

After eight months together, Dadaji announced to his disciples that he intended to give Kripalu yogic initiation, but before doing so he was to fast for 40 days on water alone in total seclusion. During his 40 days of solitude, Kripalu emerged from his room only twice a day to offer pranams respect) to Dadaji. The rest of the day he remained in utter silence, chanting mantra and meditating. These were difficult disciplines for a boy of 19, but with perseverance and encouragement from his guru, he succeeded. At the end of the 40 days Dadaji gave him yogic initiation saying, "My son, with this ancient and holy initiation I ordain you a Yogacharya (Master of Yoga). My blessing to you is that you will be the world's outstanding Yogacharya." (In the same manner, Kripalu bestowed the title of Yogi on Amrit Desai in 1969 and that of Yogacharya in 1980.)

The Disappearance Of Dadaji

A year and a quarter after Kripalu had been at the ashram, Dadaji mysteriously disappeared, leaving behind him a swirl of enigmas. Although he had many devoted disciples, none had been able to discover his true name, much less where he had come from or where he had gone. Heartbroken, Kripalu was left only with a promise: that when he finally became a swami, he and Dadaji would meet again.

Ten years later, Kripalu did renounce the world, took sannyas initiation as a swami just as Dadaji had predicted, and began the life of an itinerant monk, traveling throughout western India lecturing, writing books, and composing bhajans (songs of devotion). It was during this time that he stopped in the small village of Halol where he first encountered the young Amrit Desai. In addition to traveling the countryside teaching, Kripalu received many large donations, which, without keeping a penny for himself, he used to establish libraries, schools, temples and other institutions for the further education and spiritual enlightenment of the people of India.

All the while, his thoughts were constantly on Dadaji. Each year Kripalu visited the Himalayas for several months to immerse himself in the study of scriptures. Daily he agonized over the meaning of Dadaji's continued absence: Was he unworthy? Was his life so impure that there was no hope of ever again having the darshan (presence) of his beloved guru?

One winter evening in Rishikesh, a particularly holy place of
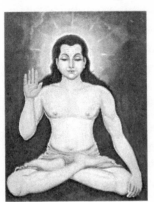
pilgrimage in the foothills of the Himalayas, an unmistakably familiar voice called to him softly, "Swami." This was the name Dadaji had used for Kripalu during their time together. Turning, Kripalu saw not the 60-year-old man he had known as Dadaji, but a beautiful youth of about 18.

"Swami, don't you recognize me?" the young man asked. The voice and demeanor were unmistakable. It was indeed his beloved Master.

As Dadaji later explained, the form Kripalu now gazed upon was his true divine body, purified by yogic fire. Kripalu became ecstatic and threw himself at his guru's feet. When he could at last speak, questions flooded forth. After spending only a short time together, Dadaji vanished.

Two long years passed. At last, Dadaji reappeared to Kripalu, this time manifesting in Kripalu's locked room. He announced to him that it was now time for Kripalu to start his yoga sadhana (intense spiritual practices). After this brief meeting, Dadaji again disappeared.

Kripalu On His Own

Guided by Dadaji, Kripalu began with six hours a day of specific pranayama practices. After this, he soon increased his meditation practices to ten hours daily, which led to his Kundalini awakening. He dedicated his life to the practice of the yoga of surrender to Kundalini Shakti, a schedule he faithfully maintained until leaving his body in 1981.

In 1955 the village of Kayavarohan invited Kripalu to speak during its holy week. By now, Kripalu was totally immersed in his sadhana, so he usually refused such invitations. However, Kayavarohan is a Maha Tirtha, a major site of pilgrimage down through the ages and the birthplace of Brahmin culture, so Kripalu accepted.

His tour of the village ended at the temple of Brahmeshwara Mahadev. There he saw a large Shivalinga of black meteoric stone with the life-size statue of a young seated yogi merged into its front. In an instant flash of transcendental insight, Kripalu recognized the full and divine truth: this was Dadaji's true form–the same form he had seen in Rishikesh, the same form he had seen again two years later.

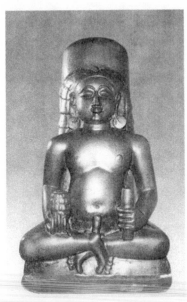

At last his guru's true identity had been revealed to him: Dadaji was none other than Lord Lakulish, the 28th incarnation of Lord Shiva himself.

As mentioned in the ancient scriptures, Lord Lakulish had incarnated in the second century BC and had revived Kayavarohan as a spiritual center of great holiness. As Kripalu's realization grew, he began to understand that Dadaji had come again in this century by borrowing the 60-year-old body of a dead sadhak (spiritual seeker) solely to train one disciple – Kripalu – to become the greatest yogi of his time.

Kripalu's realization was overwhelming. His eyes began to stream tears, his voice choked with sobs, and he began to tremble uncontrollably. He reached his hands toward the wall to steady himself and then slid slowly to the floor in grateful bliss that destiny had been so kind to him. A perfect, utter peace flooded every cell of his body.

During meditation later that day, Kripalu had visions of Kayavarohan in its former glory as it was in the time of Vishvamitra, its original founder of centuries before, and in its restored form under Lord Lakulish. In his vision, he received a divine command from Lord Lakulish and Dadaji to rebuild Kayavarohan, restoring it and making its future as glorious as its past, a spiritual center for all of India and the world.

With tearful eyes Kripalu prayed, "My Lord, your darshan has made my life sublime. I accept your commands, but I am

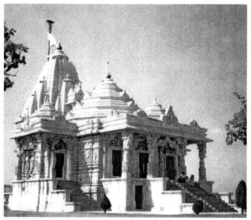

a poor and humble servant. How shall I ever be able to fulfill this gigantic task?"

And the divine answer returned, "Our chosen son, you have only to act as an instrument of divine will. The task will take care of itself." Selfless in his love, universal in his vision, and totally devoted to the spiritual uplifting of mankind, Kripalu was an example of the fully evolved master. In him was combined a blend of the rarest of qualities: the devotion of a saint, the intense dedication of one who has pursued God realization throughout a lifetime of unswerving discipline, the erudition of a brilliant scholar, and the soul of an artist. In Kripalu each of these qualities was at its zenith and it was these qualities, linked with the inspiration of divine guidance, that resulted in the restoration of Kayavarohan as a sacred mission.

Under Kripalu's guidance, the Kayavarohan Project began in earnest. Shri Kayavarohan Tirtha was finished in less than ten years and remains a standing testament to Kripalu's dedication to his life's mission. The Shivalinga representing Dadaji was installed in the central hall where devotees can view it and pay homage. The reopening ceremony of the great temple was a major event and drew a crowd of 25,000 people. Kayavarohan continues to be a mecca for the devout. It was just before the dedication of the new temple that Dadaji once again appeared briefly to Kripalu...one last time.

Sadhana–Discipline And Dedication

Since the day he took his sannyas vows, Kripalu maintained an unwavering and steadfast spiritual discipline. By the time he came to America in 1977, he had lived in seclusion and kept almost total silence for 12 years, speaking only on three annual occasions to his thousands of followers in India.

He continued his ten-hour daily meditation during his long periods of silence and during the short period of time when he addressed his American disciples every morning at the Sumneytown and Summit Station Ashrams in Pennsylvania. His lectures were full of storytelling and chanting, punctuated by his penchant for drama and comedy. Speaking in his native Gujarati, Kripalu would delight his audiences nonetheless with his presence and sweetness while Yogi Desai translated his words.

Yogi Desai had asked Kripalu numerous times to visit America and always, Kripalu had refused because it would interrupt his strict sadhana. It came as a great surprise when, in 1977, Kripalu suddenly agreed to come for a purported three-month visit. Because of the great sacrifice Kripalu was making to take this trip, Yogi Desai did everything he could to serve his guru by creating an ideal environment for him to continue his sadhana. Yogi Desai protected Kripalu from the many speaking requests that were made and was diligent about tending to Kripalu's every need so he could focus on the daily routine to which he had dedicated his entire life. Yogi Desai's wife, Mataji, who had also known Kripalu since her childhood, supported Kripalu by personally preparing and serving his meals and took care of his housekeeping needs. Because Kripalu maintained silence, he communicated by writing on a small chalkboard slate. Mataji copied down many of Kripalu's communications and kept them in her diary.

During his 12 years of silence, Bapuji communicated with his students by writing on a small chalkboard slate. Here Yogi Desai visits him in his office at Kayavarohan in 1974.

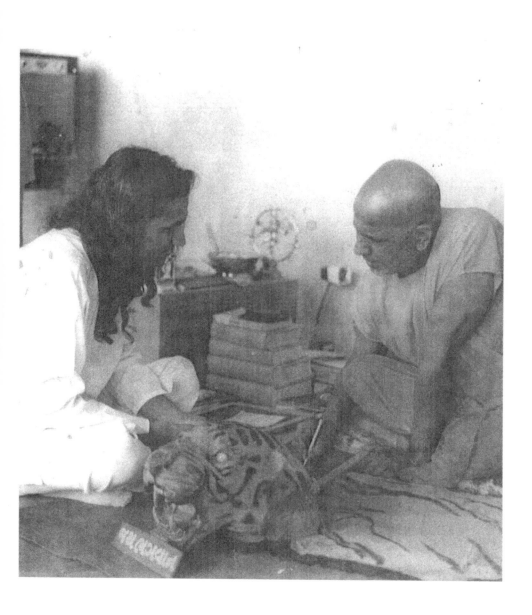

Yogi Desai grew closer to his guru during this treasured time. He had built a secluded home deep in the woods naming it Muktidham for Kripalu's visit. The name, Muktidham, means the abode of liberation. One day Kripalu called Yogi Desai close to him and said, "Today I feel that the name you gave my residence is truly fulfilled." This was a clear indication that Kripalu had reached the ultimate yogic state of complete liberation, Nirvikalpa Samadhi, the thoughtless, formless state of ultimate union—the final stage of yoga.

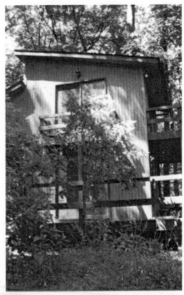

Muktidham, Sumneytown, PA

After living and practicing his sadhana at Sumneytown for 4 1/4 years, Kripalu's health began to deteriorate and he wished to return to India. Soon after his return, Kripalu peacefully left his body on December 29, 1981.

Kripalu had experienced the great secrets of Kundalini Yoga as a direct result of his own intense meditation. In turn, he personally taught them to his close disciple and spiritual son, Yogi Amrit Desai, with the blessing to bring these authentic teachings to the West.

From Master To Disciple

Amrit Desai was a boy of 15 when he first saw the man who was to become his guru. He had already developed a spiritual hunger and was immediately captivated when the young swami began to lecture. He was enraptured by Kripalu's power as a speaker, delivering powerful messages through parables. Whenever Kripalu would lecture, the young Amrit would rush to sit directly in front of him. Although Amrit was too shy to approach him, Kripalu took notice of him and recognized the qualities of a potential yogi: "I saw Amrit's inclination for the practice of yoga...I was very much pleased. In my room, I gave him a personal demonstration of my yogic practices, something I have not allowed any of my disciples to see. Amrit is the only one I ever allowed to sit in my presence during sadhana."

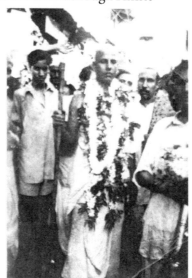

Amrit, left, at 15 with Bapuji

On that auspicious day, Amrit had silently followed Kripalu, whom he now called Bapuji, upstairs to his private meditation room. As he entered it for the first time, he sensed that it was charged with great spiritual energy. After a short prayer, Bapuji began his practices, demonstrating a remarkable flow of yogic movements and postures. Gracefully and effortlessly, he moved from one posture to the next. "Accustomed only to the traditional, methodical practice of yoga exercises, where postures are performed one at a time, I was entranced by his free-flowing demonstration," Yogi Desai remembers. "Bapuji told me that the postures are performed automatically when prana has been awakened in the body of a yogi. This is the entrance into Kundalini yoga. My young mind was unable to comprehend the magnitude of what I had seen and within a short time, I forgot the event entirely."

After studying with Bapuji for more than a decade, Amrit came to America to continue his studies as an artist in 1960. He was 29 years old, had a wife and an infant son, and was embarking on an unknown course. After arriving in Philadelphia, he struggled to adjust to American culture, going to college, finding a job and supporting his family back in India. Even then, Amrit Desai viewed his challenging situation as his dharma, his true path. Within months, he had settled into his new life and began teaching yoga on weekends.

In 1962, he had saved enough money to bring his family to America. Over the next few years, he graduated from the Philadelphia College of Art and began working as a designer while continuing to paint in his distinctive style. His work was exhibited at galleries and art shows, winning numerous awards. His life was busy, full and rewarding, but his true destiny was yet to unfold.

Turning Point–1970

Amrit Desai continued his art career, expanded his family and taught yoga for ten years after his immigration to the U.S. However, one January morning, the course of his life changed forever. In his own words, Gurudev explains the spontaneous experience that so dramatically altered his practice and teaching of yoga:

> "In 1970, I had an extraordinary experience that revealed to me a whole new dimension in the practice of yoga. One morning, I was performing my daily routine of yoga postures with my wife and two friends. However, I performed my routine with special concentration that day. A tape recording of Bapuji's yogic chants played in the background. The intonations of his voice and the gentle accompaniment of the drums stirred feelings of nostalgia and deep reverence within me. As I continued to move, I became absorbed in the rhythm of the chants. The aura of love and tranquility, which I associated so strongly with my guru filled our

32

peaceful room and brought back cherished memories of my many moments with him. Gradually I became more and more absorbed. I entered a deep meditative state, even as my body continued to move.

Suddenly as if bursting upon me like an unexpected downpour, I was flooded with energy throughout my entire being and I felt myself being irresistibly drawn into another level of consciousness. As the music dissolved far into the background, I began feeling that I was no longer the performer of the postures.

My body spontaneously entered into a flow of movements that were guided from within. These movements were accompanied by a state of ecstatic meditation deeper than anything I had ever experienced before. My movements were effortless, deeply engaging and ecstatic as if they were prompted directly from bodily urges.

My mind took a back seat. Although thoughts continued to come, they passed through my mind in slow motion, seemingly disconnected from my body's activity. I became extremely limber and elastic. The postures were emerging directly from bodily impulses unsolicited by my prior training in conventional postures. I was in awe of the new flexibility that came to me without struggle or force. My movements were no longer connected to my preprogrammed ego-mind and self-image. With no conscious effort on my part, my body was twisting and turning, flowing smoothly from one posture to the next. Some of the postures were like none I had ever seen in any yoga book.

Even though I knew I could stop the experience, I had no desire to do so. I became so absorbed in my experience, I let go of all awareness of my surroundings. I don't know how long I was in this deep ecstatic experience. As I began to become more aware of my surroundings, I found myself entering the lotus position. An intense stillness so deep that it penetrated every level of my being emanated from within me. Suddenly, an explosion of ecstasy spread through me and I became engulfed and overwhelmed by a state of complete inner bliss.

For the first time, I felt complete and total integration of body, mind, heart and spirit. All internal conflicts, doubts and impatience disappeared. It was an experience of Meditation in Motion. The movements were directly flowing from the primal wisdom of prana and consciousness.

It was truly the divine dance of Shiva and Shakti performed in the field of my body that drew me into the deepest levels of ecstasy and union. I was no longer "performing" the postures. The duality and separation of performer and performance—actor and action—dancer and dance—had disappeared. I was so absorbed in the experience I lost all sense of time. This was an experience of living in the timeless state of the present moment. I had entered a state of deep stillness in the midst of motion. This was an orgasmic experience of sacred union—of Shiva and Shakti.

Before this, I had practiced yoga for 20 years and was an experienced Hatha Yoga instructor. Even though I was extremely flexible and performed postures with great ease and understanding of the core principles of yoga, I had never entered such depth of unity. The true meaning of yoga was revealed to me experientially.

As I returned to awareness of my external surroundings, I opened my eyes to see the others mirroring my own trance-like state. My face was completely devoid of expression. My mouth was dry and I realized that I had not swallowed for a very long time. I tried to speak but words would not form. My wife and my friends had somehow been drawn into the experience with me. I found them also in deeply meditative state.

With great difficulty, they began to explain what they had felt. With deep emotion, my wife finally said, 'It didn't seem as if you were doing the postures. They looked so effortless, as if they were done without your control. They seemed almost automatic.'

Automatic. The word rang with sharp clarity in my mind, evoking the long-forgotten memory of the day when Bapuji had invited me to see a demonstration of his spiritual practices. Automatic was how I had remembered Bapuji's movements. Could my experience be similar to what Bapuji had described? Was it the result of awakened prana within me? I was in disbelief. To my knowledge, Bapuji had not taught me any specific methods that would awaken the evolutionary life energy of prana. How, then, could I, by myself, have the experience of spontaneous awakening?"

Guidance From Kripalu

"After this phenomenal gift appeared for me, I wrote to Bapuji describing what had happened. Soon, I received his reply:

My son, Amrit,
I had asked you to come here for my birthday celebration and to plan to stay with me in the

35

ashram for five days. I am now writing you the reason for this invitation.

In ancient times, the guru used to give a worthy disciple shaktipat diksha, an initiation in which the enlightened master causes pranic energy to awaken. That energy can transform the life of a disciple and lead him to the highest stage of yoga. After receiving this shaktipat diksha, the disciple would start yoga sadhana automatically, and nothing had to be taught. The practice of this would lead him to the highest spiritual consciousness.

There are only five yogis in India that I know of who can give this shaktipat diksha. When I heard this, I felt that it must be God's will. That is why I thought to prepare you to give this shaktipat diksha to your students to fulfill your worthy mission.

When you were here from June to September 1969 for higher training with me, I gave you only light shaktipat to help with your future progress. If I had given you powerful shaktipat, you would have often been disturbed in your present activities, and you would have suddenly left all your worldly work to go deeper into sadhana. But I did not give you this powerful shaktipat because it was my desire that you go into full sadhana only after you had organized your activities there.

This time I will seat you in front of me and will bestow upon you the yogic power to give shaktipat diksha to others so that this tradition may remain continuous. Remember that shaktipat does not fail even on one who cannot enter into yoga sadhana

36

with enthusiasm and peace of mind, but such a
sadhak cannot reach the highest states.

Your loving Bapuji (Kripalu)

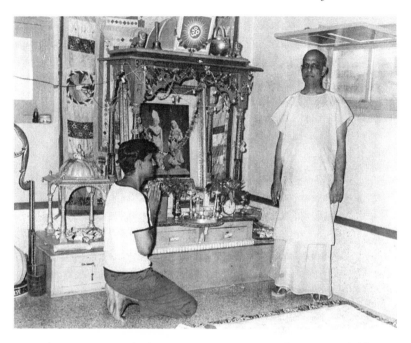

Less than two months later, on January 7, 1971, Bapuji fulfilled
his promise to his devoted disciple (pictured above). Gurudev
is one of only four of Bapuji's devotees to have received the
blessings of shaktipat diksha initiation.

The Transforming Power Of Awakened Prana

Gurudev continues his story:
  "For me this was a great revelation; I felt as if every
  experience I had ever hoped to achieve through
  yoga and meditation had happened spontaneously
  - without my trying to achieve anything. It was the
  accomplishment of divine grace.

And what a paradox for me to feel in that moment like a beginner. For 20 years I had practiced yoga faithfully. Having been awarded a doctorate of yoga by one of the supreme prelates or Shankaracharyas of India, I had all the credentials to live the rest of my life as a recognized yogi. I had established the largest yoga society in the United States at that time, having trained over 100 yoga teachers and overseeing 150 yoga classes a week. Yet this one experience was worth more to me than all those credentials combined.

To my amazement and delight, this experience recurred for me day after day. As I adopted this new, spontaneous meditative manner of practicing yoga postures, I discovered that the physical benefits I had previously derived from willful yoga exercises became greatly magnified. I fell in love with my practice even more because I was progressively entering deeper and deeper states of my being. As my mind was drawn inward, my awareness was disengaged from the external surroundings. The postures were being performed through me not by me. It was as if "I" had disappeared and had become the postures themselves.

The yoga I was now practicing took me to an expanded state of consciousness that permanently changed my life. After my initial experience, I became aware that my whole orientation to sense-objects had changed. I sensed sounds, sights, music, touch with greater depth and clarity. Sounds resonated with greater impact; colors were more vivid. Having been an artist for many years, I had always been appreciative of beauty. But now what I experienced was not just appreciation from an aesthetic or intellectual point of view, it was an ability to sense and feel the experience of beauty from an inner depth previously unknown to me.

I was able to explore, expand and experience new levels of yoga as I continued my practice. When I returned to my daily activities, I returned with greater awareness. The impact of this practice extended into the way I encountered the challenges of my life. I was able to maintain my inner balance in the midst of daily interactions. I found myself coming from a new level of spontaneity and relaxation, rather than acting from habitual behavior. My mind was freed from judgment or analysis of how things should be. In the absence of needing to impose my value system on what was, my perception became more intimate and direct. This developing sensitivity became a feedback system for me, sparking an ongoing process of self-discovery. Increasingly, I became aware of changes within myself— my posture, body language and ways of interacting with others."

Perpetual Changes

"My perceptions of other people deepened as well. It was as if I could sense and feel the more submerged aspects of people's personalities coming through their overt expression; a slight change in tone of voice or wording revealed their inner feelings to me with unusual clarity. My whole world was becoming transparent; or at least I was able to perceive things around me with much greater depth and precision. It was as if a veil had been lifted.

My yoga classes also began to change and I felt myself naturally becoming more loving and caring for my students. I realized that this unfolding of higher consciousness was mutual. As more and more of my students reported feeling these changes within themselves, it gradually became clear to me that true spiritual teachings are more profoundly communicated through direct experience.

Overnight my relationship with family and friends changed. I was still active as a parent, supportive to my wife, gardening, shopping, and laying carpet. In addition, my responsibility for my large yoga organization in Philadelphia continued. I maintained its business arrangements, paid bills, conducted yoga classes and gave seminars. Outwardly things appeared the same.

But inwardly, I experienced a shift at the core, a radical change in my values and perception of life. My pattern of relating with family and friends changed; I could no longer be the way I was. Maintaining casual friendships or attending events that were primarily social in orientation did not hold as much attraction to me, so I took part less and less in superficial conversation or social exchanges. Instead, I found myself wanting to talk about things that affected my own growth or that of others, not tangential issues. Having witnessed such depth in my practice, I could not be satisfied through contact that only touched the superficialities of life.

I also became more direct and real in my interaction with others. In retrospect I could see that I was often concerned with pleasing family and friends. If I didn't want to participate in a certain activity or eat a particular dish, I was hesitant to decline out of my wish to be kind and loving. But suddenly that part of me that tried so hard was no longer there. I discovered there was a whole new level of being kind and loving that took no effort at all. When my consciousness shifted, I saw that at some level I had been seeking other's approval as a way to validate myself. Now fearless yet loving in my communications, I had no need for validation. As a result, I could respond more directly and hear others' needs more clearly. Little by little, I began to take delight in doing things for others just for the sake of doing and in this way became wholehearted in my activities.

Detachment Arises

"At the same time, I became less and less attached to the end results. This does not mean I became aloof and withdrawn from the world around me. I simply felt more satisfied within myself, having less need to look outward for fulfillment. Not seeking personal reward in any of my customary roles as father, husband, teacher, head of an organization, I was paradoxically free to do everything with full involvement because that was simply what needed to get done.

With fewer and fewer personal agendas, my energy was suddenly freed up to genuinely respond to others. By agendas I mean behaving a certain way to get something from another person. I saw that if I had agendas, then I could never establish the level of communication I needed to create clear, loving, relationships. Neither could I be a true friend. Interacting with my wife and children, as well as students and friends enriched my process of self-discovery. From that point on, my life became dedicated to serving my higher consciousness through serving and helping others.

Even though I was in love with and totally involved with everything I did, I was paradoxically able to witness it all with great objectivity and detachment. This is the gift of the sustained practice of Amrit Yoga. The longer you engage in willful practice and encounter your own self-imposed obstacles and limitations, the more you develop witness consciousness, the ability to observe your life with objectivity and lack of struggle. When we are in love, we often lose the ability to objectively witness the person we love. There is invariably a tendency to develop blinding attachment or even addiction in the name of love. However, in this case, total involvement and love for life had no addictive component. Remaining in the witness state reduced the possibility of my developing attachment and addiction. I was in love with life, without attachment to its pleasures or fear of its pains. I felt no need to renounce pleasure because I saw that I had no compulsion or dependence upon it. I could enjoy it, but also enjoy myself in its absence as well.

" Just as I found in the postures a higher intelligence dormant within me, I also discovered a new trust in life. My newly emerging connection with the life force made my contact with the realities of life more direct. In the series of developments following my prana awakening, I was able to tap into a creative flow that brought with it a flood of sharpened awareness and understanding. Suddenly I could see deeper into the meaning of life. Every interaction and every person I met now held much greater possibility in terms of making a contribution to my own growth and learning process. I found that my experiences were all reflecting a growing consciousness of myself in transformation. Thus, I found it wasn't necessary to be an artist, a counselor, a social worker, or even a yogi. I just had to be myself. Whatever I did, the lessons emerged for my life, especially designed to release what I needed to let go of at that time. Many blocks were thus cleared in the process.

That shift in consciousness fed into a deepening trust for life; I saw that I didn't have to intervene in life's flow, but that it had its own special rhythm and purpose, which I would learn as I went along. I could stop worrying and fighting with life. I simply "did the next thing" and used that as a vehicle for expressing the creative flow that is my life. As a result, I felt empowered from my core rather than from my achievements, influence or prosperity. With that came a deep sense of fearlessness and freedom.

"I used to consider yoga a tool with which to fight the nonspiritual aspects of life. Now the distance between my ordinary life and spiritual practice was dissolving. Before that, I had ideals about how I should approach my spiritual growth. I always wondered when I would be able to begin the course of rigorous spiritual practice my guru followed. I wanted to 'get started' with a deeper practice. After this yoga experience, however, I felt so at peace with my life in whatever way it was manifesting that I stopped waiting for deep sadhana to appear. Instead I entered "meditation on the moment" and made it the prime focus of my life. Every day's experience practicing meditation in every given moment revealed countless new secrets about the meaning of life. In a way, the very experience of deep sadhana that I longed for had manifested, but in a different form than I had imagined.

All these internal shifts were a result of the awakening of prana and higher consciousness that ordinarily remain beyond the mind's grasp. It was an awakening of the core energy within me that simultaneously connected me to the core of existence as well. It was as if new internal connections were opened that allowed my external and internal lives to come into complete harmony. I myself was simply the instrument in an uninterrupted process of internal transformation.

The Mirroring Of My Transformation In Others

"The effects of my awakening were very pronounced to anyone who had known me. This experience had a profound effect, not only on my

44

family and friends, but also on my students. They began to respond to me with increased openness and sharing with me changes that had come about in their own lives as well. Those who had originally begun yoga to lose weight or learn to relax now entered into the deeper, meditative aspects of yoga and began to make surprising discoveries about themselves. Their lives radiated a new peace and happiness, which was reflected in their communication with others, their creativity and their attitude toward work. The atmosphere in the classes I taught became charged with feelings of reverence for the practice of yoga. Somehow, without having to put anything in words, my students attained depth in their practice and gratitude for the wealth of the teachings.

These changes did not happen all at once. They gradually unfolded through time. Just when I would think to myself, "Aha, I've got it!," there would be something new in store, an unending process of insights, reflections and discoveries. Above all, it opened a channel for letting go of personal controls that I had unknowingly exercised to direct my life. This became apparent after my experience of awakened prana, when rather than struggling for spiritual development, my life progressively became a flow of its own.

The Development Of Meditation In Motion

"I began to conceive of an innovative new approach to the practice of yoga, where movement and meditation can happen simultaneously and complement one another. All of my previous concepts about yoga dropped away. I had previously believed that the study of yoga and hard work would lead to deeper meditative levels. All that changed with the realization that was revealed to me that morning in 1970.

45

In keeping with Bapuji's wishes, I shaped these teachings without sacrificing their authenticity into an approach to Hatha Yoga that is eminently suited to the Western temperament. What I received from Bapuji allowed me to pioneer the teaching of Hatha Yoga as a method of achieving states of transcendental consciousness. This unique approach to Hatha Yoga is a form of Meditation in Motion that is in harmony with the ancient teachings of yoga and the Western way of life.

Since receiving Bapuji's rare and special blessing to bestow shaktipat, the sacred transmission of psychic energy that links teacher and student, many have experienced the awakening of higher consciousness. Not because of me, but because of what comes through me. My teachings come from a deep reservoir beyond my personality or sense of self. I do not consider myself a scholar or a conventional teacher of meditation or yoga. My intimate understanding of the spiritual journey is thoroughly based on my own direct experience and devotion to living in alignment with the evolutionary dimensions that Bapuji awoke in me."

V

The Core Practices of Amrit Yoga

The core practices of Amrit Yoga include: Yamas and Niyamas; Asanas; Pranayama; Witness Consciousness; and Spiritual Diet. The core practices become our daily sadhana. Sadhana is our spiritual practice that reinforces discipline toward the accomplishment of self-discovery and selfrealization. Discipline is practicing the same activity repeatedly. Sadhana is the regular or methodical practice of any one of the various embodiments of Amrit Yoga.

We become that which we repeat.

What we repeat unconsciously and habitually reinforces our unconsciousness and "bad" habits.

What we repeat consciously and habitually reinforces our "good" habits.

These good habits progressively guide us towards self-realization.

Therefore, we engage in the conscious, core practices with regularity and discipline.

Sadhana is so difficult because:

That which I am searching for is me.

That which acts as an enemy is me, and that which is attempting to get rid of the self-destructive me is also me.

I am the obstruction and I am the way.

That which obstructs is my own creation in unconsciousness.

The "I" that is the light of consciousness is hidden behind unconsciousness.

That which I am searching for is hidden behind all the false images I hold of myself.

That which remains and cannot be removed after getting rid of all that I have acquired is the real me.

VI

Amrit Yoga and the Eight-Limbed Path of Ashtanga Yoga

The Yamas and Niyamas
The Spiritual Foundation Of Yoga

The yamas and niyamas are the first two limbs of the eightfold yogic path as taught by Patanjali. These limbs are the observances and disciplines that create the spiritual foundation of both Hatha and Raja Yoga. The science of yoga is applied in our lives through the examination of our unconscious habitual patterns, beliefs and behaviors and their consequences. Observing the yamas and niyamas purifies our body, mind and heart as it also prepares us for developing the witness. The purity of body, mind and heart that we achieve from the practice of the yamas and niyamas reveals the unconscious patterns of our self-image and self-concepts.

Observance of the yamas and niyamas initiates the process of unmasking our Higher Self. The practice is not about reformation of the self-image, but about transformation and Self-discovery. If the yamas and niyamas are practiced by the separative ego with self-righteous attitudes and idealistic behaviors they turn into adapted masks. Instead of revealing the Self, such adaptations obscure the Self. Self-improvements and behavior modifications that are adapted rather then sourced from within actually set the stage for further internal conflict. Even the yamas and niyamas, if not practiced through the integrative power of the witness, can themselves become the cause of conflict. That is why in the practice of Amrit Yoga every limb must be integrated with inward focus and meditative awareness.

The purpose of the yamas and niyamas is to eliminate disturbances and conflicts that come both from within and without. They are an integral part of the posture of consciousness. The posture of consciousness is integrative; the posture of ego is separative, dualistic and disruptive to the unity of our being. Observing them allows us to see and accept ourselves where we are now while simultaneously bringing us into alignment with our intention for deepening integration and unity. Sincere practice of the yamas and niyamas eventually removes the obstacles that veil the Spirit within.

The Yamas–Observances

Ahimsa

Ahimsa's position as the first yama signifies its primary importance. It is the very seed of these basic disciplines. Ahimsa is made up of two Sanskrit terms: "a" meaning not and "himsa" meaning violent, thus "non-violence." Ahimsa is not just the absence of violence. It is seeing through the eyes of love, acceptance of self and others, kindness, tolerance, consideration, and being non-judgmental. It is called nonviolence because our limitations prevent us from understanding what true love is. But we do understand what it is not. When we let go of what it is not, what it is is spontaneously revealed. When you let go of violence, the love that is hidden behind it will emerge. Because we do not know what real love is, we automatically practice what we imagine it is. As a result, we often become the victims of our concepts of love and miss the spirit. The yogis were very wise in calling the practice of love "non-violence."

Violence can be present either in gross or subtle forms. When we are physically violent or express violent words or feelings, it is in its gross form. When we think violent thoughts, it is in its subtle form. Ahimsa must be applied to all our thoughts, words and actions.

In Amrit Yoga we practice ahimsa both on and off the yoga mat. We are attentive to our thoughts, attitudes, beliefs, spoken words and to the impact they have on ourselves and others. During the practice, we do not become aggressive, forceful or violent with our body. We remain internally aware so we do not become self-critical or self-rejecting. This is violence against ourselves. We see and accept ourselves as we are, without the need to suppress or deny our perceived shortcomings. This is the development of consciousness (non-judgmental awareness).

> "Ahimsa is the state that exists when all violence in the heart and mind have subsided. It is not something we have to acquire; it is always present and only needs to be uncovered. When one practices ahimsa, or nonviolence, one refrains from causing distress ~ in thought, word or deed ~ to any living creature, including oneself."
>
> Bapuji

Satya

Satya is truth, but to be truthful is more than not telling lies. Mahatma Gandhi said, "Truth is God, God is Truth." If we live in truth, all parts of our being–body, mind, heart and soul–our doing, thinking, feeling and being–harmoniously function with one voice. When what we feel is different from what we think and when we do something different from what we feel and think, then the conflicting aspects of our being are not being truthful with each other. This is the core of truth. When we are in Truth, we are integrated, whole, undivided and harmonious.

Thoughts, speech and actions that are unconsciously motivated emerge from unresolved conflicts. The resulting behavior represents our personal self-concepts, which are in perpetual conflict with impersonal reality. Every conflict we have with reality is the same as lying to what is. When you identify with your self-image, you are not being truthful to the all-pervading universal Self that you are.

> "We need not worry about practicing truth in speech, but merely need to delete a little untruth from the mass of untruth we usually speak."
>
> Bapuji

You cannot be truthful and honest and at the same time be identified with who you are not. In Amrit Yoga, the witness helps us move outside of all internal conflicts that exist within our self-image and brings us closer to integration with our Higher Self. Perceiving the true Self is moving beyond and transcending the pre-programmed filters of self-image and self-concepts that live in conflict and lie to the true Self.

Asteya

Asteya means non-stealing, not taking anything that does not belong to us. We must recognize that the underlying premise in all stealing, coveting or jealousy is the belief that we are not sufficient, whole or complete. We practice asteya as an affirmation that we need nothing outside of ourselves to feel complete. We are enough as we are.

> "The intention of practicing asteya is to discover that we are born divine."
>
> Yogi Amrit Desai

The root of stealing is hidden in our false assumption that we are deficient and missing something that can only be fulfilled by changing things and controlling situations outside of ourselves. The true sense of non-stealing begins with recognizing that all the deficiencies that we see in ourselves are the result of false and distorted perceptions. In reality, all deficiencies are perceived deficiencies.

When we perceive that solutions come from outside of ourselves we begin to desire what others have. This is where subtle stealing, jealousy and competition begins. Once you recognize that the source of both problems and solutions is within you, you realize that what lies within as a potential cannot be stolen, it can only be revealed, just as the Bible teaches: the kingdom of heaven is within.

When we begin our spiritual journey with this core recognition, we naturally begin to connect with the Source within and our greed and desire for what we perceive is missing is gradually eliminated. Simultaneously our connection with the infinite source of creativity, intuition, strength and wisdom is reinforced. Once you realize that the source of all solutions that you seek outside of yourself are always present within you, asteya naturally happens.

Brahmacharya

The word brahmacharya is composed of the root "char" which means to move and "brahma" which is returning to the source within—the Brahman. The literal translation of brahmacharya is to move towards Brahman, returning to the Source. The purpose of brahmacharya is to progressively move from those practices that propel us away from the Brahman. Any form of excessive sensual indulgences that deplete our vitality or life force keep us from accessing the Brahman.

Often brahmacharya is translated as celibacy. This approach is for the renunciate. For the worldly person, bramacharya is the practice of moderation and conservation of sexual and sensual energy with the intention to be in tune with Brahman–Truth, Reality, God, Higher Self, or the cultivation of the creative life force within. Thus, brahmacharya is a state of mind.

The reason for practicing bramacharya is not to create an idealistic principle that leads to guilt and self-rejection, but to cultivate and facilitate the process that leads to Selfdiscovery. We choose instead to consciously manage our sexual, sensual, mental, emotional and physical energies to enhance and assist our evolution and ultimate union with our Higher Self.

> "Brahamcharya means not indulging in sensuality, thoughts or emotions that drain your vital life force, the powerful vehicle for Self-discovery and Self-realization."
>
> Yogi Amrit Desai

As a yama, brahmacharya suggests that we cultivate thoughts, actions and emotions that increase our understanding of the conservation of shakti and its relationship to the Higher Self. Often the problem with sex is not biological but the accompanying feelings, thoughts, emotions, addictions and dependencies it brings with it. Our psychological appetites drag us into excessive indulgence in sensual pleasures. Learning how to prevent loss of vitality and prana and to direct it toward Self-discovery is at the core of brahmacharya.

To practice brahmacharya, we must be vigilant in observing how we use our energies. Again and again we must let go of all unconscious disturbances that could take us off center. With continued practice we progressively move toward the higher centers of consciousness.

Aparigraha

In Sanskrit "parigraha" means to store or accumulate with strong attachment, or to cling to firmly. The prefix "a" means not, therefore aparigraha is non-attachment, non-clinging and non-hoarding.

Aparigraha means letting go of our fear-based attachments. Fear invariably drives us towards objects of attachments as a cover-up for safety and control. Basically, all attachments are the representation of unconscious fears. Our addictions to our possessions, which we call our security, actually represent our insecurity, fear and greed. All hoarding and clinging are fear and security-based. Fear can provide us with motivation for developing resources but fear that goes into accumulating and hoarding can be released only when we become Sourceful.

As we reflect on our lives in relation to aparigraha we notice the tendency to cling to objects, people, places, thoughts, beliefs, feelings and situations. If we look deeply at our desire to cling or hoard, we can see the origins of these tendencies. We may feel strongly attracted to a person or idea and that attraction creates fear and attachment. By observing ourselves in relation to aparigraha we begin to see and feel the burden and let go of our attachments.

> "When we practice aparigraha our mechanical mental and emotional habits of attachments and fears, of attractions and repulsions, are revealed to us in the light of consciousness, providing the opportunity to let them go."
>
> Yogi Amrit Desai

We must observe both our clinging and all the fears that are attached to our clinging. When we become free from fear and attachment then aparigraha becomes a powerful tool for self-inquiry and understanding.

The Niyamas-Disciplines

Saucha

In Sanskrit the word "saucha" means purity, cleanliness, holiness, and sacredness. There are two types of purity; external or physical and internal or mental. Physical purification sanctifies our bodies, hearts and minds. Internal purification is impacted by physical purification as well as the practices of meditative awareness and self-observation. Applications of saucha on the physical level include bodily cleanliness, orderliness of our surroundings, proper diet, cleansing kriyas, pranayama, postures, mudras, mantras,right livelihood and the right practice of the yamas and niyamas. The purpose of Hatha Yoga practices is to purify the physical body, which affects the subtler energetic, mental and emotional bodies.

The physical practices of asana and pranayama, are integral in the purification process. Regular Hatha Yoga practice combined with proper diet and simplified, orderly living initiate saucha on the internal level. It is interesting to note that the word saucha means not just purity, but sacredness or holiness. With this in mind, the disciplines of purification become an act of devotion or a way of loving, respecting and taking care of ourselves.

Saucha is not an imposed discipline or a rule we must obey. It is practiced from a place of insightful understanding and awareness. The embodied purity and sacredness reflects itself in the way we experience ourselves and in our interactions with the world around us. It spiritualizes and transforms every expression and expands our view of life with compassion, love and selfless service.

The internal aspect of saucha focuses on awareness of our toxic emotions, thoughts and attitudes, especially our habit of indulging in negative thinking such as self-criticism, competition, jealousy, judgments or self-defeating perceptions and emotions.

> "If you realized the destructive impact of self-defeating thoughts and toxic emotions, you would immediately let them go."
>
> Yogi Amrit Desai

In Amrit Yoga, our intention is to heal our body, clear our mind and purify our heart, and bring them into alignment with our highest potential, not by suppression or denial, but by acceptance, trust and faith. To awaken our inborn divinity we must continually let go of that which we are not. Saucha happens when we are the witness. As we cease to nourish our thoughts by identifying with them, fighting with them, denying them or suppressing them, they die of starvation. We are left with the awareness of our inherent innocence, purity and oneness with the Source.

Santosha

Santosha means contentment. It is the ability to tolerate and digest all the opposing experiences of duality with the equanimity of an ocean. Even though all rivers flood into the ocean, it remains unperturbed, allowing all waters, whether still or rushing, to enter its vastness. Similarly, the yogi lives in the world, yet remains content, despite the ebbs and flows of life.

Santosha is the unconditional state of being. Being free from addictions and fears creates the objective state of observation of the witness. Such objective observation is impersonal without personal preferences for or against what is present. Impersonal reality has no commitment to adjust to our personal fears and addictions.

Learning to remain established in the changeless state of the witness embraces all opposing experiences that constantly alternate with ups and downs, success and failure, happiness and unhappiness, pleasure and pain. The movement of duality is circular. Santosha is like the hub of the wheel that remains a constant center around which all opposing experiences move. That is why the world is described as Samsara Chakra, the wheel of life. Santosha is the direct result of remaining a changeless witness to all the opposing experiences of the phenomenal world. Changelessness is the state of our being, of our soul.

When we are aligned with santosha, we are not anxious or impatient to get anywhere. There is no worry or fear, and therefore we are fully present and content with being in the present. Santosha creates entry into the dimension of grace and fulfillment that comes not from doing something to get somewhere but from being in the undivided, timeless state of living in the present. Being in the now does not require any doing or desire for change.

> "When we are not seeking excitement, life becomes exciting in a very deep way. It is joy without excitement. Then, when excitement comes, it is not like a rushing river but like deep still water-there is hardly any movement on the surface."
>
> Yogi Amrit Desai

Santosha gives us the ability to receive happiness without attachment or addiction. Santosha has nowhere to go in order to be fulfilled. If it is not fulfilled in the now, it cannot be fulfilled in the future either. When I, who consider myself to be deficient now, arrive in the future, regardless of what I have achieved, I still arrive with my sense of deficiency intact. Here the problem is not of having more, it is the problem of not feeling that I am enough. If there is such a thing as eternal damnation this is it. What I have, cannot ever replace who I believe I am.

It is not a problem of hard work, greater effort or more skills. It is a problem of lack of knowledge of who I really am. Once I believe I am deficient, greed for more can drive me forever without ever having any possibility of driving out the sense of incompleteness I have assumed. False assumptions can never be solved by acquisitions. My belief of myself survives all achievements. Only knowledge of the true Self can take us out of the self-imposed bondage of the selfimage.

The witness is the only way to dismantle the invisible walls we construct to protect the self-image that separates us from the true Self.

Santosha is an adventurous journey that demands everything you have to arrive in the here and now. Santosha does not demand security; it demands fearlessness, faith and trust. In reality, everything that comes in the future happens only in the now. When your attention is divided and fragmented between now and the future, your creativity, efficiency and ability to function effectively is greatly reduced. Being present is productive, not passive. When you are totally present, your ability to enjoy what you are doing happens naturally all along the way rather than at the end of a miserable journey. Santosha is a journey from moment to moment. It is not driven by fear and anxiety. Only in the absence of fear and anxiety can we live in the present with love, faith and trust. This creates compassion for the world rather than frustration with the world.

Compassion is the most powerful way to serve humanity. When motivated by fear or frustration, even the search for peace turns into war.

Tapas

Tapas is the generating of light and heat, as in the process of smelting or making finer metals. Just as fire purifies gold, restraint or discipline purifies the body, mind and heart of the seeker. Thus, tapas is the spiritual heat that is generated when we go through the process of letting go of our self-image so that the true Self may begin to surface.

Whenever we sense threats to our self-image, our instinct of self-preservation reacts with the fight or flight reflex. Even if it is only a perceived threat, we react as if it were real. All survival-based reactions, whether for the protection of the physical self or for the protection of the self-image, are both unconscious and instinctive.

In yoga our intention is to move from our unconscious, instinctive reactions to a conscious response to what is. If you fight your unconscious reactions it only feeds your selfimage. When you are in the witness, you detect your unconscious reactions and do not act out of reaction.
Unconscious reaction invariably manifests as fight or flight. When you are compulsively driven either by fight or flight, simply relax, breathe and let go. Create a space between the point of impact that ignites your reaction and the reactive action. This space is the window of transformation. It is in this window of transformation that we experience tapas. The only way to create this space is to remain witness to our first reaction. When there is no space between impact and action, it is reaction, not conscious response. All reactions are kneejerk impulses that do not leave us the opportunity to correct our conditioned misperceptions.

The witness prevents us from being thrown into instinctive, unconscious reactions. Every time you choose not to act out your reactions you are starving your self-image. If you fight it, you feed it. If you run from it, you feed it. Only when you remain witness to it can you starve it. The starving is the dying process of the self-image, which creates the spiritual heat of tapas. Out of the ashes of the burning of the self-image arises the phoenix of the true Self.

But the self-image does not give up so easily. The ego will try to prevent tapas by finding different ways to release the pain rather then resolve the source of the pain. This only creates a temporary escape. We run away from facing reality and from taking full responsibility for the pain we are experiencing.

In order to prevent pain our ego takes one or more of the following measures to avoid addressing the real source of the problem:

℥ fights to save our self-image
℥ finds that we are too weak to resist and runs away
℥ blames someone else
℥ shames ourselves

The dying process of the self-image engages the ego with the same instinctive reactions it uses to protect itself from threats to physical survival, health and well being. This tapas is the alchemy where the unconscious is turned into consciousness and the preprogrammed self-image is transformed into the Self.

In Amrit Yoga postures are practiced with the highest intention to create tapas. It is focused on burning away psychosomatic toxins and blockages. We deliberately stoke the inner fire that leads us toward purification of the mind, body and heart. Our intention is to let go of the selfconcepts and impurities that obscure our recognition of the light. By practicing tapas we become increasingly more identified with the light of consciousness as it glows ever brighter through our bodies, hearts and minds.

"To purify the mind, the average seeker should begin by attempting to accomplish tapas of the body. Tapas of speech and tapas of the mind will automatically follow."

Bapuji

Swadhyaya

Swadhyaya is composed of two words: "swa" meaning Atman and "adhyaya" meaning to study; that is, to study the Atman. We practice swadhyaya to know our true Self. One of the cornerstones of Amrit Yoga is swadhyaya–selfobservation, introspection and self-inquiry, where unconscious beliefs, self-concepts, resistances, reactions emotions, and self- rejections are clearly exposed in the light of consciousness. Swadhyaya is non-judgmental selfobservation through witness consciousness, a systematic way of disassociating from our self-image. Just as the clouds move away and the light of the sun is revealed, when the mask of the self-image is removed, the light of the Self shines through.

The central focus of Amrit Yoga is meditative awareness, which is the most powerful tool you have to loosen the grip of identification of the self-image. To be released from the unconsciousness that separates you from the true Self, you must step back from the filters imposed by the self-image. The most direct way to accomplish this is through swadhyaya. The witness creates an opening by unmasking self-concepts that actively intercept and distort your perception of reality, helping you let go of past conditioning and everything else that is holding you back.

In witness, you are unbiased, clear and objective, detached from past conditioning and future expectations. This helps to solve problems and resolve conflicts with the reality that is revealed in the present. Impersonal reality is the source of all solutions. As you grow in witness, your personal biases grow weaker.

As the witness starves the self-image, the Higher Self begins to reveal itself. Amrit Yoga is a process of unmasking the Self. To successfully perform this process we must experientially study the Self not only through the formal discipline of yoga but also through every interaction in our life.

Ishvara Pranidhana

Ishvara Pranidhana means dedicating all the results and consequences of our actions to God. When we surrender the results of everything we do, our actions are also dedicated in the service of God. Letting go of the end results requires complete faith and the absence of fear or need to control, which comes from the unconscious, separative forces of the ego-driven self-image.

All actions that are performed with separative consciousness are performed with an attachment to the end result. Such attachment is the opposite of surrender to God. In the practice of Amrit Yoga, mindful meditative focus helps us disengage from our personal biases. Each time we learn to let go of fears and attachments, we automatically surrender. With an attitude of surrendering the results, our actions lose their capacity to produce emotional reactions and mental agitations.
The sense of success and failure is suffered only when we are caught in personal likes and dislikes, addictions and fears. When we surrender our preferences to God, we remain unattached to either success or failure.

Being disengaged from success and failure frees our mind from agitation and our heart from emotional reaction. Energy and attention freed up from such unconscious preoccupations becomes available to focus on whatever we are doing in the present. Giving up attachment to the end result, the mind becomes alert, tranquil and attentive. All of its faculties are activated to function effectively, optimally and creatively.

> ᎕ When our mind is peaceful and our body is relaxed, we remain free from preoccupations with anxiety, impatience and fears.
> ᎕ When we are fully present and totally engaged in whatever we are doing, it automatically becomes a deeply fulfilling, satisfying experience.

63

ଔ When we are disengaged from attachment to our
   dreams, we are not driven by impatience, self-doubt and
   stress.
ଔ When we are present, fulfillment happens all along the
   way rather than at the end.
ଔ When our heart is free from fear and agitation, we
   become more insightful, intuitive and perceptive.

We must recognize that all the consequences of our actions are
essentially the function of the law of karma. By letting go of
the end results of your actions, you discontinue the chain of
creating new karma that comes with personal likes and dislikes.
When you surrender your personal addictions and fears, you are
also free from the consequences of success and failure.

Only love and faith in God can empower us to live without
fear and the need to control. Such love and dedication to God
gives us the trust that allows us to live in freedom from anxiety
and stress of the unknown future. Love, trust and faith must
first arise in one's heart before it can possibly be surrendered
to the Lord. The Bhagavad Gita says, "The Lord abides in the
heart regions of all beings. To surrender to the Lord means to
dedicate one's every thought, word and deed to the Lord." In
yoga, the abode of God is within.

> "Only a lit lamp can light an unlit lamp. If we perform
> one hundred actions for ourselves every day, can't
> we perform one or two actions for our beloved Lord
> who is our true relative and well-wisher? After all,
> actions dedicated to ourselves are useless actions
> and bring only pain; but actions dedicated to the
> Lord are genuine actions and bring true happiness."
> Bapuji

Physical Disciplines

Asanas

Physical yoga postures are used as an entry point to the true practice of yoga. Stage I of Amrit Yoga is willful practice, with the main focus on learning the postures correctly but without force or aggression. This means working through personal fears, physical inhibitions and self-concepts. Willful practice does not violate or override the wisdom of the body. Instead it works with the body consciously and deliberately.

Enter each posture with awareness and respect for the body. Focusing on proper form and alignment does not mean forcing yourself to achieve perfection of the final form. Instead, remain focused on performing the posture to the best of your ability. It is the deliberate practice of correct form, not the perfection of the posture that provides the maximum benefits. Your journey begins from where you are. It cannot begin from where you are not. Remember to:

 ∞ Follow precision, alignment and attention to details.
 ∞ Make your movements slow, focused and intentional to help you move through areas of your body that you might otherwise avoid.
 ∞ Pay attention to what your body can and cannot do, rather than judge or compare your performance with others.
 ∞ Accept the limitations in your body.
 ∞ Drop internal resistance when you discover your physical limitations. Breathe, relax and let go of stress and holding as you encounter the inhibitions in your body.
 ∞ Relax and remain more attentive and focused on what is happening within you.

Postures or asanas are the specific physical positions of the body used in Hatha Yoga as a foundation for the spiritual disciplines of Raja Yoga. When the physical discipline is isolated from its mental and spiritual components, it loses the integrative core of yoga. This is why Amrit Yoga uses asanas in combination with physical, mental and spiritual disciplines.

Patanjali's *Yoga Sutras* describe asanas as having two essential qualities: sthira and sukha. Sthira means steadiness or alertness. Sukha is the ability to remain relaxed, comfortable and composed. Both qualities should be equally present not just in the physical posture but must also be an integral part of the mental and emotional postures that accompany it. The physical experience can be the beginning stage of sthira and sukha, but without the mental and emotional bodies being an integral part of that steadiness, it is not complete. Sukha applies not only to the physical postures, but also to psychic postures, those uncomfortable and awkward "postures" we must hold in our everyday life. The practice of yoga develops inner strength so that when you are surrounded by a hurricane, you remain centered, relaxed and composed, as if you are in the eye of a storm.

When the physical, mental and emotional bodies are steady and composed, it is called "the posture of consciousness," where all bodies are harmoniously integrated in the posture of yoga. The steadiness of the body cannot occur independently of the mental and emotional states that regulate it.

When the central focus of asana is physical, there is no way to fulfill the core intention of the practice of yoga, which aspires to bring the body, mind, heart, and soul into harmonious unity. In Amrit Yoga, the primary focus is learning to perform the postures with awareness of the body's limitations, steady, relaxed breathing, and precision and attention to detail, combined with mindful meditative attention. This leads to prana awakening, the stage prior to Kundalini Yoga. The final stage of Amrit Yoga happens when the prana-shakti that carries out all the evolutionary activities in our body is awakened and the spontaneous practice of asanas occurs. It is a state of dynamic meditation where you experience stillness in motion.

Pranayama

The word pranayama is composed of "prana" meaning breath or life force and "ayama," meaning to extend. Pranayama is the mastery and management of prana. The intention is to both increase the retention of prana and prevent the misuse of prana. It is also used as an independent discipline for detoxification of the physical body to release blockages from the psychic bodies. It is a powerful means of awakening prana-shakti and nadi shuddhi, clearing the channels in both the physical body and the subtle bodies.

Pranayama also refers to breath techniques used to move into deeper and subtler layers of tension in the physical postures. It is also used to keep the mind steady as we encounter psychic, mental and emotional boundaries such as fear, resistance, criticism or doubt. When we breathe, relax and let go, our attention is disengaged from reaction and we can easily focus on the details of the posture and awareness of sensation. Breath now becomes a way to establish witness consciousness and to remain fully present in the experience of now.

Through the practice of yoga asana and pranayama we discover the relationship between the breath, the body and the mind. We can see that stress in the body or fear in the mind instantly alters our breathing patterns. Consciously changing our breathing releases the conflicting unconscious forces that keep us from being relaxed and present, both during our practice and in our daily lives.

The Universal Prana

In a larger sense, Prana (distinguished as Prana with a capital P) is the divine life force. It is the eternal energy or shakti of God. It is omnipresent, omnipotent and omniscient. It is the pure life energy that intelligently regulates every process of the universe. It is the neutral indestructible life force that accounts for the rhythm and harmony by which all things and beings in the universe are born, exist, dissolve and evolve again.

The entire world goes through the cycle of birth and death, involution and evolution, under the precise laws of Prana. Through Prana, we are connected to everything that exists. This principle is the basis for the yogi's understanding that there is a profound interaction and connection between the body and the mind, between a person and the world around them, and between the physical, mental and spiritual forces. This energy is also known as the Holy Spirit, the handmaiden of the Lord, divine Shakti, Kundalini and Chi. Yogis believe that through in-depth understanding and use of this energy, God can be realized and experienced directly. It is the extensive teaching on the relationship of Prana to the physical body, energy body, mental and emotional body, and the applied use of this energy, that adds the spiritual dimension to the practice of Amrit Yoga.

Prana and the Wisdom of the Body

Prana flows through the nerve currents of our body and carries out millions of intricate life-giving processes with precise order and intelligence. This wisdom of the life force that works within our body unceasingly is at the core of all life-giving functions. Science calls it an "involuntary" system; yoga calls it an "intelligent" system. We never had to learn how to breathe, circulate our blood, digest our food, eliminate toxins, or heal our bodies because the life force of prana, with its unparalleled intelligence, carries out all such complex processes day and night from birth to death. This life force is our constant unfailing companion and wisest friend, our protective Divine Mother, Shakti. There is no force or person capable of providing us with the protection and sustenance we continuously receive from prana.

The harmonious functioning of the body and prana depends upon the mind's cooperation since the mind is the controlling and processing station for all the inner needs of the body. The condition of the mind strongly impacts the condition of the body and the functioning of the five senses, as well as the prana that fuels it. If the mind is confused, prana is confused. When the mind is restless, prana is restless. This is why in Amrit Yoga, we give highest priority to the internal focus which regulates the restlessness of mind and emotional reactions that continuously create disturbances in the body.

When your prana is unconsciously used in self-destructive ways, it creates the psychological and emotional stress we call self-rejection and guilt, which sometimes turns into blame and shame. These are all the manifestations of our inability to recognize the power of prana and its relationship to our body, mind, heart and soul. The knowledge of prana's role in every expression and experience of life gives us deep insight into how to use all the levels of our being harmoniously to connect with the infinite source of the soul.

Prana mimics the mind and assumes the patterns that are created in the mind and emotions. The patterning of prana directly corresponds to the mental and emotional conditions that control them. The moment we operate from unconscious emotional reactions or self-destructive thoughts, prana begins to carry out whatever thoughts or emotions we are assuming. Consequently if the mind is disturbed, it will automatically disturb prana in the body. Prana is the fuel for our physical actions, sensual perceptions, thoughts and emotions. As we expend our energy in indecision, fear, doubt, impatience and emotionally charged mental dialogues and images, we lose a tremendous amount of life force. Once we learn how to harness these forces through Amrit Yoga we can learn to dismantle this self-destructive use of prana, which is essentially an enemy-in-residence. It works against us day and night. However, by turning it into our most intimate friend, we can rebuild our health, restore our youthful vitality and reverse the aging process.

Prana's Relationship to Breath

When we speak of prana (with a lower case 'p'), it can be either prana as the life force or prana as the breath. Breath is the most fundamental, visible link to life. It connects the body to the mind and the mind to the body. Breath is a bridge between the body-mind because it is subtler than the body and grosser than the mind. Breath, combined with consciousness, has the added impact of harmonizing the conflicting unconscious forces that keep you from being relaxed and focused during your yoga practice and in your daily life.

Breath can eliminate stress not only in the body, but also stress that is continually introduced by thoughts and emotions. Use the breath to manage your internal psychic posture as well as your external physical posture. Breath is psychosomatic; it integrates, modifies and orchestrates the body-mind experience. Pain in the body is held in the muscles and joints. In the mind, fear of being hurt adds defensive muscle resistance, which is the body in reaction. So when you are performing a yoga posture, you encounter two types of pain:

α3 Pain that is already lodged in the body.
α3 Pain that is held in unconscious memories of the past that manifests as fear in the mind.

When there is fear in the mind, it is reflected as protective tension in the body. Notice how your breath changes to accommodate physical, mental and emotional stress.

To shift out of reaction to fear or pain, you must deliberately shift out of your protective breathing pattern. Let go of either holding the breath or breathing erratically. Return to slow, deliberate rhythmic breathing to simultaneously help you release both fear and pain from resistance. Changing your breathing pattern is an integral part of the willful practice. It is effectively used whenever you find yourself fearful, resistant, stressful or in discomfort. When this happens, there is an unconscious tendency to hold the breath. This represents fear and an attempt to prevent pain.

In reality, holding the breath is another way of holding and feeding your old patterns. It supports unconscious fears and resistances that you face in your body-mind. Conscious use of the breath allows you to shift out of old habits and replace them with new awareness.

When you encounter resistance in your body, notice how it shows up in your breath. You may instinctively hold your breath or breathe erratically to cope with the discomfort. This also happens in life situations. When life puts you in an emotionally uncomfortable posture (when you are caught in fear, insecurity, resentment or emotional reaction), your psychic body is placed in a yoga posture. Resistance manifests as emotional reaction caused by fear of loss of control in a given situation. You are facing a psychological boundary whether you are in a physical posture or a psychic posture. Whether you are on a yoga mat or in life, you are in a yoga posture. Maintain internal focus and meditative awareness to release the fear, resistance and emotional reactions that you encounter.

Prana and Spirit

Breath is also the link between the physical body and the soul. The prana that is linked to breath is biological prana; the Prana that is linked to the soul is the Spirit-Prana. Spirit is the source of life; breath is the visible link between the body and the soul. When the soul leaves the body, it is called a corpse. In the absence of Spirit-Prana, the body cannot assimilate prana through breath. Soul is the primary source of life that is at the core of the life-giving breath that sustains our health and well being.

Breath is bio-energy. Soul is spirit-energy. Bio-energy is Shakti and spirit is Shiva. This explains how pranayama in Amrit Yoga is not only breath work but also a powerful tool for awakening the evolutionary power of prana and reconnecting us with our soul. When breath is combined with inward focus and the integrative power of the witness, you are not just breathing air and oxygen, but Prana that awakens the potential inborn divinity of the soul. This is what transforms ordinary breathing exercises into a sacred tool for realizing your divine potential.

> "Prana is a wise and protecting energy. It knows fully well how best to carry out its involuntary functions so as to bring comfort and purification to the seeker. The seeker remains a witness to all the spontaneous activities of Prana, which occur during the meditation and receives all its guidance from Atman-Soul through the aid of prana energy. This is the aspect of God within us."
>
> Bapuji

Considerations for pranayama:
- The inhalation and exhalation should be slow and smooth. Avoid erratic movements.
- When you hold the breath, hold comfortably. In order

72

to allow the exhalation to be smooth and long, do not strain during the holding.

ও During the posture, keep your attention on the sensation of the breath in the body.

ও Inward focus and awareness of sensation during pranayama will bring you to the higher stages of Amrit Yoga.

Techniques of pranayama:
I. The Complete Yogic Breath

1. The complete yogic breath is done in either a crossed legged position or in shavasana (corpse pose), lying flat on the back with the legs about a foot apart and arms by the side with palms up. In either position, relax completely. Exhale fully.

2. Inhale deeply through your nose. Allow your relaxed stomach to expand like an inflated balloon.

3. Exhale through the nose and contract your stomach muscles until the diaphragm expands and presses upward into the thoracic cavity under the ribs.

4. Continue breathing until you have established a natural rhythm. Notice your abdomen rise and fall.

5. Repeat this abdominal breathing five to ten times.

6. After one week of practice, continue to breathe abdominally, but add the following: after filling your lower lungs, concentrate on filling first your middle lungs, and then your upper lungs. As you exhale, first deflate your upper lungs, then your middle lungs, and then deflate the abdomen. Make your breath steady and rhythmic, like a wave rising and flowing in, and then flowing out again. This is the complete yogic breath.

Benefits of the Complete Yogic Breath:

Relaxes the entire body and nervous system, particularly the abdominal region where we hold so many tensions and anxieties. Relaxes the heart, reducing blood pressure. Massages the abdomen, toning the organs, stimulating digestion, regulating intestinal activity and elimination. Provides relief from respiratory problems.

Regular practice increases the amount of air taken in with each inhalation, using more of the lungs, resulting in more oxygen intake from each breath, and hence slower respiration. This creates calmness in the body and increased clarity of the mind.

II. Ujjayi–Sounding Breath

1. Sit with spine elongated and erect or lie comfortably in shavasana (corpse pose) for the ujjayi breath.
2. Inhale through your nose, drawing your breath in slowly. Contract the back of your throat slightly as if making an "ahhh" sound, but with the mouth closed. This will create a slight hissing sound at the back of the throat as the air passes over the windpipe. Contracting the back of the throat also lets you regulate the flow of your breath, thereby allowing you to prolong the inhalation and exhalation. As you continue with the slow inhalation, let your abdomen relax and expand as in the complete yogic breath.
3. Continue to contract the back of the throat slightly as if making an "eeee" sound, with the mouth closed, while you exhale. Exhale as you slowly pull the abdomen in and up to fully empty your lungs. Control the flow of your breath. Let it be long and slow.
4. Continue to inhale and exhale in this way.

III. Kapalabhati

In kapalabhati, the exhalation is forced, the inhalation

spontaneous. There is a split second of retention after each exhalation.

1. Exhale vigorously through the nose: at the same time push in your abdomen; then allow the inhalation to happen passively by relaxing your abdomen. This is one round.
2. Repeat in a steady rhythmic series of exhalations according to your capacity. Emphasize the exhalation each time.
3. Variation: Instead of using both nostrils you may alternate nostrils, closing off right nostril then left nostril with alternate exhalations.

Benefits of Kapalabhati:

Cleanses and purifies the entire respiratory system by forcing air from the extremities of the lungs. Clears the mind and improves concentration by increasing the amount of oxygen in the system.

Kapalabhati can be practiced at the end of each round of abdominal pumps to quickly regain natural breathing. This practice is forceful and is strenuous for those with weak lungs and fragile constitutions. It is contraindicated for those with ear infections or glaucoma, and for those with high blood pressure. If your nose begins to bleed, or your ears ache or throb, discontinue use for a while.

IV. Anulom Viloma – Alternate Nostril Breath

In this breathing technique, inhale through one nostril, retain the breath, then exhale through the other nostril in a 1:4:2 ratio. As an example, we will use the count 2:8:4.

1. Sit comfortably. Place your right hand in the Vishnu mudra (tuck index and middle fingers into palm). Bring your hand close to your nostrils. Use the thumb to close off the right nostril and the third and fourth fingers to close off the left nostril.

2. Close the right nostril with your thumb and breathe in through the left nostril to the count of two.
3. Hold the breath, closing both nostrils to the count of eight.
4. Keep the left nostril closed with your third and fourth fingers. Breathe out through the right nostril to the count of four.
5. Keep the left nostril closed and breathe in through the right nostril to the count of two.
6. Hold the breath, closing both nostrils to the count of eight.
7. Keep the right nostril closed with your thumb and breathe out through the left nostril to the count of four. The above procedure constitutes one round of Anulom Viloma.

Benefits of Anulom Viloma:

Anulom Viloma plays a powerful role in awakening prana. It restores a balanced flow of prana to the body. It has a calming, stilling, balancing effect on the mind, which helps one to more readily enter meditation.

V. Nadi Shodhana

This technique is the same as Anulom Viloma without the holding. Breathe in through one nostril and exhale through the opposite. Practice this technique before advancing to Anulom Viloma.

"Pranayamas are extremely useful for the spiritual seeker. In fact, there is no better penance than the practices of pranayama through which impurities of the mind are removed and real knowledge dawns. As the dross of metals like gold is removed by heating them in the fire, so also the dirt of all the senses is removed by the practice of pranayama."

Bapuji

Mental Disciplines

Pratyahara

Pratyahara means withdrawing attention from internal distractions as well as external disturbances that enter the mind through the five senses. During the practice of asanas, remain relaxed and aware, slow down movements, and synchronize the breath with movement to create pratyahara. This is the development of meditative awareness in the practice of Amrit Yoga. When thoughts, feelings or emotions come, let them pass by without judgment, analysis or concern. Making no mental comment either for or against the experience, return your attention to the breath. Simply be the observer, unperturbed by whatever is occurring, either from within or without.

Pratyahara, in combination with dharana (concentration) and dhyana (meditation), create a state of inward focus. In Amrit Yoga, pratyahara is introduced in Stage I, more deeply explored in Stage II through holding the posture, and in Stage III it evolves into the practice of Meditation in Motion. Pratyahara is a prerequisite of dharana, but when we are engaged in concentration, pratyahara naturally happens. They are highly complementary.

Dharana

Pratyahara is the preliminary stage for dharana (concentration). Unless you have learned to withdraw your attention from disturbances you cannot establish yourself in concentration because pratyahara and dharana are not practiced separately but simultaneously. The mental disciplines of pratyahara and dharana are the preparations for dhyana.

Pratyahara and dharana cannot be practiced successfully without the presence of meditative awareness (dhyana). When you encounter distractions such as physical resistances and mental and emotional reactions, your concentration will invariably be disturbed. What helps you to come back is mindful meditative awareness.

The intention of dharana is to focus your attention in one direction to train the restless mind to stay fully present. When the mind is in a state of dharana, pratyahara automatically occurs. While in pratyahara or dharana, we cannot be distracted by internal emotional reactions or resistances that come up when we encounter our physical, mental or emotional inhibitions.

In Stage II of Amrit Yoga we consciously hold the posture and focus on the bodily sensations that accompany the holding. Bodily sensations become the object of concentration, while we dispassionately observe the thoughts and feelings that arise. The more we develop concentration in our practice the more subtle and refined our awareness becomes. We become more attuned to the subtle urges of the body. When the body is released from prolonged holding, the flow of prana becomes more intense and more tangible. We are then able to follow the guidance of prana as it speaks to us through the urges and impulses that come through the body. As a result of pratyahara and dharana, we can more easily bring the mind into greater harmony with the workings of prana. This mind-body attunement is the gateway to Stage III—surrender to prana.

Spiritual Disciplines

Dhyana

When our flow of concentration is uninterrupted and we are absorbed with whatever we are concentrating upon, then we naturally move toward meditation. Dhyana (meditation) is a natural continuation or deepening of dharana (concentration). Dharana must precede dhyana because the mind must be focused before meditation can occur. This is why all techniques of meditation are, in one way or another, the techniques of concentration that help you slip into the meditative state.

In Stage II and III of Amrit Yoga, we concentrate on the sensations in the physical and subtler energetic bodies while remaining firmly established in witness consciousness. This is also present in Stage I during the second half of the posture. This process leads to the final stage of final stage of union–Samadhi.

In dhyana we observe the fluctuations of thoughts and emotions with choiceless awareness. This allows the inner wisdom of the body to carry out prana-guided movements without the intervention of mental or emotional distractions and disturbances. When the movements are guided by the evolutionary wisdom of awakened prana, it becomes Meditation in Motion.

As we surrender to prana we automatically let go of the preprogrammed karmic conditioning that we identify with as our self-image. We disengage from the inner conflicts that are the cause of all of our suffering. We let go of anything that would interfere with our connection to our inner Source.

In Amrit Yoga the state of dhyana is where the deep inner transformation of our practice occurs. We move from

79

identifying with our self-limiting concepts into the realm of oneness, wholeness and integration that is the heart of yoga. Yoga is the experience of union, where the doer and the doing are no longer separate. The doer disappears into doing, the dancer disappears into the dance, and the performer disappears into the performance.

The Final Experience of Yoga

Samadhi

The literal translation of samadhi is ecstasy and bliss, or to bring together, to merge. In samadhi we become so absorbed in the object of meditation that our mind becomes one with it. Our identity–name, history, relations, and all selfconcepts–completely disappear. Samadhi is a state of grace. The ancient scripture, Gheranda-Samhita, speaks of Samadhi as a great yoga, which is acquired through good fortune and through the grace and kindness of one's teacher and by virtue of one's devotion.

Samadhi emerges naturally as the result of pratyahara, dharana and dhyana. As the conflicting forces of body, mind and spirit are harnessed and harmonized, you enter an ecstatic experience that is deeply absorbing, relaxing and fulfilling. When you are guided by the inner wisdom of prana, energy floods through your entire being. You merge into the infinite ocean of cosmic consciousness. The earlier stage of samadhi occurs with thought. Later it develops into a thought-less, transcendental state.

Once this state is experienced, even for an instant, there is a strong desire to return to it. Each time you experience this silent ecstasy it becomes easier and easier to return there and to remain longer. Samadhi is the essence of the Amrit Yoga experience. It is the realization of the ultimate state of complete bliss, integration and pure being.

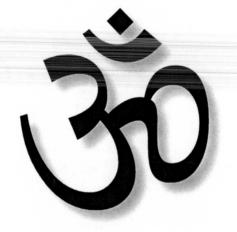

VII

The Three Stages of Amrit Yoga

Although Amrit Yoga is divided into three distinct stages, you learn to integrate all limbs of Ashtanga Yoga from the very beginning. In Stage I, attention is on the practice of physical postures. Still you begin to cultivate the internal focus that includes pratyahara and dharana. In the later stages, you deepen your practice by integrating pratyahara, dharana and dhyana, the components of Raja Yoga.

The focus of the practice is learning to give undivided attention to details along with internal awareness, which keeps you free from distractions such as frustrations with your own performance, fear of hurt and pain, self-criticism, comparison and competition. In Stage II, when you have already learned how to perform the posture correctly, your attention is no longer engaged in learning the technique. Now you can focus predominant attention on internal bodily sensations.

As you enter Stage II, you progressively begin to observe all physical sensations—comforts and discomforts, mental disturbances and emotional reactions—as objects of your meditative awareness. This form of distancing from your own body, mind and emotions allows you to enter the process of self-study and self-observation that leads to Self-discovery.

After you have practiced Stage II sufficiently enough to create nadi shuddhi (deep purification of the body, mind and heart), prana awakens. When that happens, you enter Stage III, the final stage of Meditation in Motion.

Stage I: Willful Practice

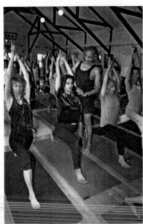

At the first level of yoga practice, traditional Hatha Yoga postures are performed with attention to correct form using press points and energetic extensions. These techniques will help you overcome physical inhibitions as well as protect you from injuries. Correct form also requires you to interact with areas of the body that you ordinarily tend to compromise, ignore or avoid.

Yogi Desai with his daughter, Kamini, who is a senior Amrit Yoga teacher and contributor to this book.

Postures are always performed with respect to your body's limitations. There is no struggle or force in the integrative approach to the practice. Every obstacle is overcome with deliberate action. Unconscious fight or flight reactions are replaced by conscious effort. In willful practice, there is effort with an absence of force. Unconscious effort in the practice of postures only yields mechanical benefits. Struggle and force, or fight or flight reactions, are manifestations of unconscious fears. Conscious effort is not fear-based. Nothing of inner value can be attained without the accompanying inward focus and awareness.

Your body is not an enemy to be overcome. Your practice is not a fight against your body; rather it is intended to establish a loving relationship with your body. Struggle and force are born of an unconscious approach to the practice and breed inner conflict. Conflict and unconsciousness live together. The presence of one brings on the presence of the other. One of the purposes of yoga is to eradicate unconscious forces and replace them with the integrative spirit of consciousness.

84

This stage draws on the strength of our willpower exercised with consciousness. The purpose of Stage I is to unblock the subtle channels (nadis) of the body. This preparation is necessary for the awakening of prana in the following stages.

Willful practice is a conscious victory over unconscious inhibitions and limitations and guides us toward greater freedom, which brings health, vitality, and flexibility. The aim is not perfection but intention that sets direction.

Stage I Focus Points:

Precision of Postures

Entry into each posture is performed with great attention to detail. The movements are slow and intentional. By deliberately slowing down, you allow yourself to notice intrusions of the mind. When combined with breath, the willful postures generate a powerful flow of energy in the body and the nervous system. In willful practice, three things are directed: effort, attention and energy.

Breath Control

Managing the breath results in deep purification and strengthening of the physical body and mind. (See section on Pranayama for specific techniques.) There is a tendency to hold the breath when you feel strained. Instead, when you feel discomfort—relax and breathe deeply. Changing your breath pattern changes your experience. Regulating your breath will help you cross physical, mental and emotional boundaries, taking you to a deeper level in a relaxed rather than a forced way.

Notice how deep breathing helps you let go of the defensive tensions that keep you from moving deeper into the subtler levels of the posture. Remember to breathe in coordination with your movements. Deliberately slow down your movements to match your breath, and use your breath to let go of subtle resistances and reactions. Breath is the link that connects the mind with the body and the body with the mind.

Deliberate, not Forceful

The aim of willful practice is not to achieve a "perfect" posture. You receive the benefits of yoga by being mindful of proper form and correct alignment to prevent injury. It maximizes the impact of the posture regardless of your flexibility. Attention is switched from forcing yourself into a position to consciously and deliberately putting the body into the posture with great respect toward the body's ability. At this point, you shift from struggling to attain a pose to remaining relaxed and respectful of your body's limitations. You will begin to notice areas of tension, pain or strain. Your mind will keep trying to interject: "This is too hard." "My back hurts." "You're so lazy, you know you can do better." When that happens, dismiss the mind's intrusion and redirect your attention to the details of the posture.

There is a saying, "No pain, no gain." Pain without consciousness is simply pain. It produces more resistance and expands the original scope of pain. Pain consciously endured brings freedom from pain. Willful practice trains you to endure and encounter pain deliberately. You will find freedom from pain, not with resistance, but by joyously encountering it with an intention to go beyond it.

Inward Focus

Inward focus in Stage I is about withdrawing from all the usual distractions that keep us from focusing on the correct form of the postures. The most common distractions in the earliest stage are ego-based, such as fear, self-criticism, comparison and competition with others. This form of self-judgment creates internal conflict, which is counter to the integrative spirit of yoga. With mindful awareness, ideas of comparison and criticism evaporate. Fear and resistance disintegrate, liberating you from all judgments about yourself and your practice.

Acceptance of Limitations

When you accept the limitations that you encounter in your body while performing postures, you initiate the first step in the process of Self-discovery. When you release internal resistance, resentment and reaction to your boundaries, your body naturally relaxes. An instant relaxation comes over you like a healing wave. When you accept everything that you discover about yourself and resist nothing, then all unconscious conflicting forces dissolve into the all-embracing light of awareness.

Transition Time-The Second Half of the Posture
(refer to the next section for an in-depth discussion on the significance of this aspect of practice)

The transition time is a period of reflection and reintegration. It can be used each time you transition from one posture to another or at the end of several postures. Your integrative process is most active in this interim period. No matter how well you have performed the first half of the posture, it is not complete without conscious integration of the energies that have been released during the posture. It is the experience of deep absorption and integration. Let your attention be totally engaged and absorbed in the flood of energy that is released during the postures. Feel the sensations of the released energy throughout your body and bring your attention to the Third Eye. This will integrate all of the energies released from the shadow self and transform them into light.

Stage II: Will And Surrender

Stage II is a dynamic blending of willful practice and surrender. Using the impetus of will power, you will now take the skills you have acquired in willful practice to a new level through extended holding without force or expectations. The holding is steady and mentally relaxed, not driven or ambitious. Guided by intention, give yourself the permission to experience any feelings, emotions or thoughts that occur during the holding. Prolonged holding, combined with internal focus and meditative awareness, supports your intention to enter the deeper layers of tension consciously. The more you remain internally focused and conscious, the more penetrating your awareness will be to release the subtler (psychic) layers of tension.

You are now moving into the next dimension, which is *letting it happen* rather than *making it happen*. At this stage, the application of rigid form and technique can be an inhibition. Once you have practiced willful postures and developed your inner strength, you gradually shift to the practice of letting the wisdom of the body choreograph the movements. This is called surrender to prana.

You are learning to shift the authority from your mind to prana. Instead of your movements being conducted willfully, you are letting the impulses of prana guide your movements from within. Let go of your confinement to the form, as learned in Stage 1. That which is an asset in the willful stage becomes a liability in the practice of surrender. In willful practice, making it happen is the core value, and in the practice of surrender, letting it happen is the core value. In surrender, the positions of the body are developed by the intelligence of prana in direct response to inner promptings.

Intention takes you deeper toward the integrative experience of your body, mind, heart and soul. You are able to move from addressing the physical boundaries to the unconscious boundaries of the mental and emotional bodies. Stage II is based on the principle of complementary balance between will and surrender. This stage naturally matures into the third stage.

Stage II Focus Points:

Prolonged Holding

Holding the posture for an extended period allows you to enter into the deeper layers of tension held in the body. This actively releases physical, mental and emotional blocks that are not accessible when you do not consciously choose to enter deeper levels of the posture. Even though you are performing a physical posture, in reality, you are holding the posture of consciousness.

The posture of consciousness accesses all tensions held not only in the physical body but in the mental and emotional bodies as well. At all times, keep your undivided attention on bodily sensations. Consciously enter and penetrate the subtle layers. You will invariably uncover unresolved hurtful experiences and fears that are stored in your unconscious and muscle memory. The instinctive "fight or flight" response will manifest. Whichever way it manifests, breathe into the sensation it brings, relax and let go, observing it, but not reacting to it. The resulting inner experience is so powerful and engrossing that by maintaining the posture, you can easily guide yourself into absorption and deep concentration.

Mindful Meditative Awareness

In Stage II, you begin to merge with the more subtle principles of yoga. Prolonged holding initiates the practice of the higher limbs of yoga–pratyahara, the withdrawal of outgoing attention; dharana, concentration; and dhyana, meditation.

Learn to free your attention from seductive unconscious forces that distract you from within and without (pratyahara). You achieve that by always bringing your attention back to bodily sensations (dharana). In order to anchor your unbroken stream of attention to your bodily sensations, you must embrace all opposing experiences of comfort and discomfort, pleasure and pain; your personal likes and dislikes, attractions and repulsions, with non-participative choiceless awareness (dhyana). Mindful meditative awareness is the doorway to integrative yoga. By letting go of resistances on the surface, you are able to delve into the deeper levels of what is truly happening at subtler levels, where the karmic blockages are held.

Although karmic blockages are held in the subtle bodies they are revealed in the physical body. During prolonged holding, you come face to face with your karmic blockages—the painful experiences and emotional traumas from the past. Now is your opportunity to encounter them and release them, allowing the energy of prana to heal unresolved karma. Karmic blockages are what hold you back and prevent you from realizing your spiritual potential. Developing this state of subtle penetrating awareness disengages you from your self-image and reconnects you with the Self that you are. It is in this stage that you develop the therapeutic and evolutionary dimension of Amrit Yoga.

Bodily Sensations

Amrit Yoga is a journey from the head to the heart. In Stage II, you learn to move from your thinking (head) center into your feeling (heart) center. The mind is ordinarily and consistently drifting away and getting caught in internal reactions. Focusing on sensations helps you to harness those internal disturbances. You learn to withdraw your attention from distractions and conflicts by focusing an unbroken stream of attention exclusively on bodily sensations. Your attention to bodily sensations is not only focused during the practice of postures but continues even after the completion of the posture.

When you harness your attention through focusing on bodily sensations, extraneous disruptive energetic forces cease to work against you. Internal attention to bodily felt sensations puts you in touch with the subtle mysterious workings of the life force that were previously beyond your range of perception. This form of increased sensitivity gives you greater mastery over unconscious forces that, unknown to you, work against you. Unconscious reactions and physical stress are the major impediments to perceiving the workings of the energy fields. The moment you are deeply relaxed and become conscious without condemnation for the weakness that is revealed, your sensitivity and subtler perceptions are wide open. This increased sensitivity to bodily sensation, with mindful meditative attention initiates the integrative process of body, mind and heart.

The Transition from Willful to Surrender

Willfully prolonging the posture creates a build-up of energy. When you come out of the posture, the release of dammed-up energy results in deep relaxation. If you relax into the experience, your body's impulses will naturally guide you into a complementary pose. This guidance comes directly from the wisdom of your prana-body. Stay with the sensations, listening to your body. This allows you to recognize what your body needs and respond to its guidance. The impulses arise directly from the body not from conscious will. Surrender to the inner guidance. Assume different positions as directed by the wisdom emerging directly from your body.

Stage III: Surrender

Stage III is a formless yoga practice that drops any use of techniques learned from outside authority. Confinement to the formal practice is now totally abandoned. The movements of the body are spontaneously guided by the awakened wisdom of prana in the body. It is an intuitive flow of movements guided from within that generates the positions in response to the inner needs of the body. Conventional postures will appear but they are not willfully introduced. You no longer choose willfully what to do or what to avoid. You observe that

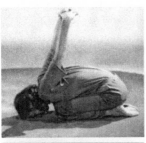

the movements are chosen by the intelligence of the body. The postures may or may not be traditional.

Deep relaxation awakens prana from its involuntary functions and takes it to an evolutionary level. The same intelligence that carries out the intricate life-giving functions in our body now begins to tailor yoga postures, pranayamas and other movements to release the blockages on the subtler karmic levels that cannot be accessed through willful practice.

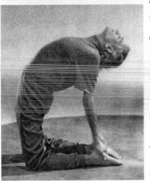

The meaning of surrender is not submission of your higher power. Instead it is letting go of the self-destructive unconscious forces that sabotage your higher Self.

Stage III Has No Focus Points:

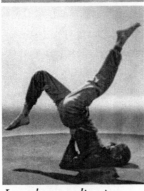

In a deep meditative state, Yogi Desai performs a series of asanas he calls the posture flow.

The first two stages detoxify the body and cleanse your nerve channels. All the regenerative processes of the body are accelerated. You experience increased flexibility, strength and endurance and regain youthful vitality. These are all the signs of nadi shuddhi. This leads to the awakening of prana. As a result, you will be more in touch with your body and its promptings, impulses, urges and guidance that direct your movements from within. When you are guided from within, your movements are no longer confined to formal or prelearned postures. The movements are tailored and prioritized to precisely meet the inner needs.

In willful practice you must know the particular situation you are working on in order to consciously direct your attention and action to resolve it. You know where the problems are because you are interacting with those that have already surfaced and are recognizable. In surrender, however, you have no conscious knowledge of the subtle blockages that exist within. You give complete freedom to the higher intelligence of prana to diagnose and direct a particular posture, breathing technique, lock, mudra or cleansing kriya to directly target the problem.

The purification of the body through dedicated practice of the prior two stages prepares you to trust the intelligence of the body. Spontaneous movements manifest and breathing patterns are regulated from within. You are no longer confined to the challenges of the body willfully as you were in the earlier two stages. You are using physical postures as a spiritual vehicle to explore and experience deeper levels of consciousness.

Witness consciousness now has grown into the full-fledged experience of unconditional surrender to prana. As a result, you experience new possibilities for the unfolding of spiritual powers. Staying at the physical level limits you to the first three chakras—the third stage takes you to the higher integrative centers of consciousness.

Stage III is where we let go of being "the doer." Thus when you allow your postures and movements to emerge from within, unedited by your mind, the wisdom of the body choreographs the positions, sequence and holding time to precisely meet your own body's needs. Such moments that originate directly from beyond the mind are spontaneous, effortless and deeply engaging.

When we surrender our will to the wisdom of the body and allow its impulses to guide our movements, it is meditation in motion.

"During Kundalini Yoga meditation, actions are performed without any conscious will. The question arises, "How does this happen?" The answer is that the entire physical functioning of the body works under the control of the mind, but the mind itself does not carry out any activities. It orders prana to follow its commands. During Kundalini Yoga meditation, the mind's control over the body is lifted. As a result, prana becomes free. Prana then becomes a guardian and operator of the body. Without paying any attention to the orders of the mind, prana makes the body perform various activities in order to protect and purify it. Physical organs perform actions without one's will during meditation. One begins to performs various asanas, pranayama, and mudras without having previously learned them."

Bapuji

VIII

The Second Half of the Posture

Postures and the Release of Prana

The period that follows the actual performance of the posture is the second half of the posture. The posture of consciousness does not stop with the completion of the physical posture. It extends into the transition time. No matter how brief the interval, no matter how short the transition time, anchor your undivided total attention to fully feel the flood of energy released by the posture. Feel the presence of the released energy in the form of sensations in your body. After feeling the sensations fully in your body, draw your attention to the Third Eye.

The Integrative Center of the Third Eye

All of the energy that has been released from the tensions in your emotional or physical blocks will be carried instantly by your attention to the Third Eye. It is in the Third Eye that the energies of the shadow self and psychic blocks are transformed through an integrative process that converts darkness into light, duality into unity. The Third Eye is the integrative center where dualities lose their conflicting forces and become integrated, harmonious and whole.

The transitions or spaces between each asana are just as important as the formal postures themselves. In releasing the posture, remain attentive to every movement and bodily sensation. Every time you finish the posture allow yourself to enter into the celebration of deep release. Being engaged in the bodily sensations of the released energy is the most absorbing experience of the mind naturally merging and melting into the energy body.

There are two levels of integration:
- ᛓ the first level is the release of blocked psychosomatic energies;
- ᛓ the second level is integration of the released energies through the Third Eye.

Most yoga practices only engage themselves in the release of energy. Guiding the released energy to its integrative state in the Third Eye is seldom recognized. As a result, a crucial, integrative experience of yoga is not fully encompassed.

The integrative process that begins by releasing stress- and fear-bound energies into the body during the yoga posture continues to move towards deeper integration during the interim period when you may think you have already finished the posture. Keep your attention deeply engaged in the sensations that are felt in the body not only during the postures but also after the release of the posture. During the posture you are unblocking the unconscious psychosomatic forces and during the transition time you are integrating those forces by transforming them from darkness into light.

Prana Mimics the Mind

This merging of the mental and energy bodies takes place when the mind is no longer the carrier of its unconscious programming. The prana body mimics and follows all the conscious and unconscious activities of the mental or emotional body. When the mental or emotional body is in confusion, hesitation, doubt or impatience it is instantly reflected as inhibition in the prana body. This prevents prana from freely carrying out all the life-giving, healing and regenerative processes.

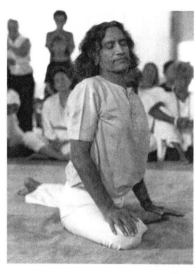

Amrit Yoga provides the techniques and tools to disengage these energies from our unconscious. Our pranic energy is held hostage by compulsive, unconscious forces that will not easily release it. To disengage prana from unconscious forces, Amrit Yoga uses the powerful spiritual tool of inward focus and meditative awareness to systematically reconnect with the Source.

When the mental and emotional bodies deeply integrate into the energy body, all of the distractions that are ordinarily present in the waking state disappear. Each time your mind releases its control over prana, prana energy acts with greater strength and freedom to carry out internal healing at a much higher and accelerated rate. This is the process of freeing prana from the unconscious forces that actively work through the medium of the mental and emotional bodies. This is the meaning of surrendering our will to prana. Once you learn how to surrender to sensations, you will be able to enter the deeper-level experience of ecstasy and unity of yoga.

Remember: The first part of the posture that you willfully perform releases the blocked energies. The second part is entry into a state of non-doing, where you simply receive the full impact of released energy as it is felt in the form of sensations.

Healing Prana Goes Where it is Needed

When prana is disengaged from the psychosomatic blocks during postures, the energy that is released is no longer contaminated or charged by the personalized, preprogrammed conditionings of our self-concepts. This energy (prana) that is disengaged from the self-concepts assumes the original primal purity of universal intelligence. This pure energy perceives clearly without personal distortions and is then available to be used deliberately and willfully for surrender. When our energy body is purified then we can naturally live in beginner's mind. The more energy we transform from unconscious psychosomatic blocks to the Third Eye the more we become self-sourcing, self-confident, creative, intuitive, insightful and objective in our perceptions and directions in life.

During the postures, if your attention is scattered and disturbed by your personal preprogrammed patterns of mental and emotional reactions, then your energy remains engaged in old karmic patterns. Erasing these karmic patterns is the real work of yoga; letting go of the old conditioned past that lives in the unconscious. This integrative process continues throughout the entire practice of Amrit Yoga in either the performance of the posture, holding the posture or in the transition in between. For this integrative process to be complete, you must remain in mindful, meditative awareness to all the subtle sensations that accompany each and every movement.

Staying in the feeling center requires acute vigilance to recognize any mental or emotional interference that draws away your attention. In order to keep the internal focus total and undivided, you must remain in your feeling center without being caught by personal biases and conditioned reactions.

For you to enter this level of deep integration you must remain inwardly focused, deeply feeling the energy flowing and flooding in different areas of your body. You're simply observing the impact of the movements, stretches, holding and releasing of the posture. Every time you come out of the posture, use inward focus to observe the impact of released energies. This energy invariably follows your attention and also increases the impact of

98

the released energies. If you miss it, no matter how well you have performed the first part, you have gone only half way.

Remaining in the Witness

When you remain in this non-participative, choiceless witness you will be able to disengage from mental and emotional distortions that disturb your ability to live totally and fully in your bodily sensations. The more you remain witness to your sensations the more you will find that the prana body will be released from the distorting influences of the mental and emotional bodies. This is the process of purifying your prana body. As a result, you will find the contaminations that are imparted by the mental and emotional bodies into the prana body are progressively separated. The practice of Amrit Yoga helps you return to the innate, primal intelligence of prana. This process of returning is what Christ meant when he said, "Unless ye be like children again, ye cannot enter the kingdom of heaven." In Buddhism the same state of consciousness is expressed by the term "beginner's mind." Again, remaining witness to the internal workings of prana automatically allows your released prana to feed your higher Self rather then your emotional or mental bodies.

All of our preprogrammed beliefs, personal biases, attractions and repulsions, addictions and fears, form the body of our self-image that we also know as our persona or mask. In order to maintain, nurture and protect this mask from being exposed, our unconscious, survival instinct engages the life force of prana to support and sustain that self-image. This is how the distorting influences of the self-image weaken the healing power of prana. When the self-image protects itself, it draws on the life force of prana. As a result, prana becomes distorted and fails to fulfill its innate evolutionary process to lead us toward the higher centers of consciousness.

The entire process of the practice of Amrit Yoga is designed to free the prana body by disassociating it from the unconscious, preprogrammed self-image, personal biases and belief systems that limit the freedom of the healing power of prana to serve as an evolutionary agent of the higher Self.

Bhagavad Gita-Chapter V, Shloka 11: "The yogi, abandoning attachment, performs actions with the body, the mind, the intellect and the senses, only for self-purification."

IX

The Mental and Spiritual Disciplines of Patanjali's Yoga Sutras as Integrated in Amrit Yoga

The self merges into Self through the medium of the meditative practice of asanas.

In Amrit Yoga, asana is the vehicle, and the objective of the practice of asanas is to progressively enter deeper levels through pratyahara, dharana and dhyana, and merge into the ultimate experience of yoga–samadhi.

Each limb of Ashtanga or Eight-limbed Yoga, is designed to reintegrate the scattered forces of the physical, mental and emotional bodies. As you develop the three aspects of one-pointedness (pratyahara, dharana, dhyana), you enter ever-deeper and subtler layers of experiencing the reality of the universal source of all that is. When you are connected to this source, returning to it again and again, your mind automatically functions in perfect harmony with impersonal reality.

The deeper the integration, the greater the illumination of the Higher Self. This progressive one-pointedness and absorption is movement toward the unified field of consciousness. This is the journey from personal to impersonal, from unreality to reality, from untruth to truth; from darkness to light, from time-bound consciousness to the timeless state of being.

Asatoma sad gamaya	Lead me from the unreal to the real.
Tamasoma jyotir gamaya	Lead me from the darkness to the light.
Mryitorma amritama gamaya	Lead me from time-bound consciousness to the timeless state of being.

Prayer from The Upanishads

Yogas citta-vritti-nirodhah (Chapter I, Shloka 2)
Yoga is the stilling of the modifications of the mind.

The basic philosophy and the intention of the practice of all disciplines of yoga are revealed in this sutra. It represents both the fundamental purpose and the ultimate experience of yoga. If you fail to understand this core concept, you miss the heart of yoga.

What we seek through the practice of yoga is the union of the individual soul with the supreme soul–God. It is a transition and transformation from the separative personal being to oneness with the impersonal being, from time-bound bodymind consciousness to the timeless state of being.

Through its identification with subjective conditioned reality, the individual soul has become separated from the omnipresent universal reality. The soul undergoes involution and separation from the Source. The purpose of yoga is to enter the evolutionary cycle of integration toward reunion with the Source.

The mind does not exist as a thing. It is not something substantial. It exists only as a process. It is an activity, such as dancing. When you stop dancing, where does the dance go?

Dance is not an object; it is an activity. Thinking is also an activity. The moment you stop thinking, the mind stops. We use the word "mind," which appears as an object but is really a process. It is an activity that can start, speed up, become distracted, slow down or stop altogether.

In deep sleep, the mind comes to a stop. But in sleep, you are unconscious. Through the practice of yogic disciplines, you can consciously transcend the mental limitations that operate within the time-space, subject-object, cause-effect dimension. When you transcend time, you transcend the mind. When the mind stops, you enter the timeless state of transcendental unity in yoga. So Patanjali writes: *Yoga is the stilling of the modifications of the mind.*

The mind, with its modifications, is the carrier of the mask of our preprogrammed personality. It is this mask that keeps the individual soul from experiencing union with the cosmic soul. The mind is the medium through which we enter the time-space dimension. The spiritual potential of the soul becomes identified with the personality that is trapped in the dimension of relativity and duality.

"Stilling the modifications of the mind" means transcending the illusion of relativity and duality. It means going beyond the time-bound consciousness that creates self-deception of glorious tomorrows and conditioned memories of the past that prevent us from being fully alive in the present.

As mental agitation diminishes, your body becomes progressively more and more relaxed. Your movements become effortless, spontaneous and self-fulfilling. You lose the sense of time. Your movements are guided not by your egomind but by the higher, non-mental intelligence of prana.

The inherent awakened wisdom of prana guides the movements of the body while the mind remains a silent observer. Your mental modifications stop; the performer egomind is silent and prana is active.

Mental activities are like clouds. They come, they go; they form, they dissipate; they appear, they disappear. When thoughts disappear, your being manifests into the full glory of the vast, limitless sky of infinite possibilities. This state of "letting it happen" rather than "making it happen" is the paradoxical union of yoga, where doing becomes being. You are in dynamic stillness, where modifications of the mind stop and yet the body continues to move, directed by the nonmental intelligence of prana. This is Meditation in Motion.

When you are fully established in the witness, all mental activity, its movement in the past and the future, memory and hope, identification with personality and objects, all disappear. You enter the timeless state of ecstasy and unity. In the witness, there is no identification with objects or modifications of the mind. This transcendental state liberates you from the limited field of the body-mind dimension. The mind naturally calms down and eventually enters deep stillness. In the absence of identification with all modifications of the mind, you are in the world, but not of the world. You operate in the world, yet you live beyond it.

Sva-visayasamprayoge citta-svarupanukara ivendriyanam pratyaharah (Chapter II, Shloka 54)
Pratyahara, the fifth limb of Ashtanga Yoga, is the withdrawal of the mind from sense-objects.

Ordinarily, our sense-perception is connected not only to the five senses (sight, sound, touch, taste and smell), but also to the mind. We are continuously bombarded by many sensual impacts from the outside world but we tend to only be attentive to those that we are attracted to or repulsed by. The clock ticks continually, but without attention, we do not hear it. The mind rides on the senses. Senses are the vehicles of the mind, but the mind is the master of the senses. In the absence of attention, senses cannot be in contact with the object of the mind.

What occupies our mind and creates mental and emotional disturbance can be divided into three major categories:

1. constantly changing impressions received from the external world that bombard the five physical senses
2. memories and images of past experiences
3. anticipation, expectations and images of the future

The first kind of disturbance comes from the outside world, but reactions to them come from within. All incoming essential impressions are not received as they really are. Often what we experience instead is our preprogrammed reaction to sense-perceptions. Pratyahara cannot be isolated as a disturbance from outside because all disturbances are fundamentally the result of pre-programmed reactions of our personal likes and dislikes. Numbers 2 and 3 are personal pre-programmed reactions to number 1.

Distractions and unwanted intrusions prevent us from maintaining our inward focus. However, when any senseperception is outside of our personal attractions or repulsions, our mind automatically ignores it. Any time we are not particularly focusing our attention on something specific, we discover our mind is overflowing with mental images, projections, interpretations and fantasies. When conditions that demand attention are absent, mental and emotional restlessness returns. Predominant unresolved thoughts and feelings of anger, fear, hurt and pain take over. This is the why we attempt to ignore such feelings by keeping ourselves preoccupied with superficial activities.

When we want to practice concentration of mind, our preprogrammed attractions and repulsions toward different senseobjects create disturbance. Pratyahara is about cultivating our abilities of withdrawing from distractions both from within and without that keep us from moving into deeper levels of concentration, meditation and samadhi.

When you consciously relax different parts of the body, you withdraw outgoing attention, which gives you the ability to gather scattered energies and fragmented mental and emotional forces. This establishes the proper conditions for the next limb, concentration (dharana), as well as the later stages of yoga.

Personally distorted reactions are completely independent of objective reality. Distorted reactions that arise on the mental plane can be transformed into pure and direct perception of reality through concentration and meditation. Thus, the practice of pratyahara, dharana and dhyana are deeply related and interdependent. You cannot remove the distracting impact of any sense-perception without detached attention, which distances us from the object of perception. When our entire being functions in perfect harmony with the universal source, all the forces of nature and our inner source automatically help us reach the higher level of health and fulfillment in every area of our lives. As you enter higher states of integration, your whole life starts unfolding toward deeper levels of satisfaction, fulfillment and contentment.

How does this work? When the internal source of ongoing conflicts is removed, the entire nervous system and the energy field of an individual become free from stress. The body enters a spontaneous healing process, the mind becomes calm and emotional disturbances are automatically resolved. As a result, you live in love, harmony and peace in restful awareness. These conditions are the foundation for accessing higher sources of creativity, intuitive insights, and protection from within that help you work through all crises you encounter in life with equanimity.

Desa-bandhas cittasya dharana. (Chapter III, Shloka 1)
Concentration (dharana), the sixth limb, is the confining of the mind within a limited mental area (the object of concentration).

This sutra defines the meaning of concentration (dharana). Pratyahara is withdrawing attention from outward distractions; dharana is directing attention to the object of concentration. In the practice of Amrit Yoga, dharana is central to the mental discipline that is integrated with the physical discipline of Hatha Yoga. After you have practiced withdrawing from external and internal disturbances, you have simultaneously created the facility to focus your attention on a given object. Dharana is confined within the area defined as its object of concentration. Within the object of dharana, there is a moving center that allows you to navigate within the fixed boundary of the intended field of concentration.

When you reach a deeper level of concentration you become one with the essential nature of the object. Concentration in the yogic system allows you to enter the core of the object that you are concentrating upon and reveal its invisible and subtle essence, which is inaccessible through ordinary concentration.

Yogic concentration differs from ordinary concentration. Ordinary concentration can be tainted by personality and personal biases. Attention narrowed by pain, fear, jealousy or competition is not concentration. These are instinctive unconscious forces or inborn urges, which automatically demand our attention when we feel insecure, unsafe or fearful. Narrowed attention is desperately driven by unconscious forces of fear or addiction. Such concentration takes you deeper into old conditioned unconscious patterns and develops a constricted sense of self.

For example, someone working in business, sports, music or dance can be very focused and attentive to his field. One can attain a great degree of concentration driven by personal biases, attachments, addictions, competition and jealousy. These reactions are all separative, self-seeking orientations to concentration. When you are in competition, caught in jealousy, extreme happiness or fear, the mind does become very focused. These are motivated instinctively and controlled unconsciously and involuntarily. In yoga, concentration is deliberately directed to remove any involuntary, unconscious distraction.

When you learn the more conscious level of concentration, it becomes expansive, particularly if it is combined with choiceless awareness. This helps you identify restrictive, narrow concentration and turn it into expansive, detached attention. Concentration is preparation for deeper integration, which matures into meditation. It is used as a vehicle to release you from buried karmic patterns held in the unconscious, subtle bodies.

Conscious attention creates a new opening where you can shift out of old self-concepts, personal biases and fears into impersonal universal reality. Consciously induced concentration creates resolution out of conflicts; response out of reaction; light out of darkness; integration out of fragmentation; and an expanded sense of self out of a constricted sense of self.

So in yogic concentration, the mind is confined within an established territory, which allows limited freedom of movement. In Amrit Yoga, the object of concentration is unresolved memories accumulated and stored in your body. This is initially felt in the form of mental and emotional reactions to the sensations of pleasure and pain. These are preprogrammed memory fears (resistances) of old hurts.

Here the term bodily sensation excludes personal reactions to the sensations, which can distract you from concentration. Yogic concentration implies detached attention and inward focus.

Sensations may range from comfort to discomfort, pleasure to pain, from tension to relaxation, yet the mind must stay fixed on the object of concentration, which means embracing all sensations unconditionally. Here the object of concentration is restricted to experiencing pure bodily sensations without labels or judgments. Comments that arise from personally conditioned attractions and repulsions, such as "I like it" or "I don't like it" put you into personal reaction rather than pure experience.

Because the sensations are moving from one part of the body to another and cover an array of feeling, this concentration is not confined to a single point but moves through the range of sensations. At no time does it leave the object of concentration. If the mind moves away from the object of concentration (bodily sensation) and becomes connected to an irrelevant object, concentration is broken.

Every time your mental concentration is broken from its connection to sensation, it is a distraction and you must instantly bring it back. The main intention for the practitioner is to learn how to reduce the frequency of such interruptions and progressively eliminate distractions. As the depth of absorption increases into the present moment's feelings and sensations in the body, the frequency of disturbances lessens.

Concentration demands alert awareness and internally focused attention. As you progressively eliminate vague and blurred impressions of what you are experiencing in the body and learn to replace them with sharply defined bodily felt perceptions, your concentration becomes more focused.

Detached attention allows you to reconnect with the dormant dimension of your being. The light of choiceless awareness and detached attention heals the divided self and all the internal conflicts, stress and suffering it causes. It acts as a beacon of light that dispels the darkness and reveals the divine Self.

Tatra pratyayaikatanata dhyanam.
(Chapter III, Shloka 2)
Uninterrupted flow of the mind toward the object chosen for meditation is contemplation (dhyana).

As you begin to enter the process and practice of meditation, mental and emotional interruptions become less frequent. When you succeed in eliminating such distractions completely, you spontaneously enter dhyana.

If the continuity of attention is occasionally broken, it remains concentration (dharana) When concentration matures into uninterrupted continuity of attention, it becomes meditation (dhyana). In dhyana you become deeply merged into your object of attention. When you are totally absorbed, you are vibrating in resonance with what is. This reveals the inherent secrets that are invisible through ordinary consciousness.

Meditation means complete concentration with an unbroken stream of attention to the object. It completely occupies the mind without any distraction from within or without.

In dhyana, all physical, mental and emotional fluctuations come into perfect resonance and resolution. Along with the attainment of this inner silence and stillness simultaneously arises the ability to be in direct resonance with present reality so completely that the full range of its inherent mysteries blossoms from within. Every human suffering that comes from avidya (ignorance of reality) is resolved when the light of reality begins to shine forth from within. Meditation leads us to direct experience of the universal impersonal reality which is ultimate resolution and freedom from all human suffering.

Tad evarthamatra-nirbhasam svarupa-sunyam iva samadhih
(Chapter III, Shloka 3)
When the citta (the mind) becomes absorbed in that which is the reality and is unaware of separateness or the personal self, this is contemplation or samadhi.

Samadhi is entry into the impersonal world of the universal presence of reality, where you have broken all the limitations of perceptions bound by the self-image. Time-bound consciousness comes from identification with your body, mind, emotions and opinions. The experience of union lies beyond our individually conditioned mundane world. This union unlocks the door to the world of omnipresent reality. What keeps us from direct intuitive knowledge of reality is our self-image, self-concepts or subjectivity that separates us from the object and hides the reality and freedom we are seeking. At this stage, meditation helps us transcend all physical, mental and emotional barriers that come from identification with our self-image. This reveals the secret of hidden guidance, protection, and creativity of the Higher Self. When you merge into the experience, something is revealed. It is neither logical nor rational; it is spontaneous.

Samadhi goes through many different stages of deepening experience. In the earlier stage of concentration, the object is separate from the subject. In meditation, there is a progressive movement toward subject-object integration.

The earlier stages serve as preparation and later culminate into the final experience of union. As you enter the preliminary

111

stage of samadhi, it is known as savikalpa samadhi, where the meditator experiences bliss, but is aware of the object of experience. The first stage of samadhi is very much like arriving at the gates of direct realization of our true nature, but unless the depth of complete absorption is reached, the essence escapes our grasp. To reach this state, the separation of subject-object must be eliminated. One must be so totally absorbed in the object of meditation that all boundaries of the body-mind and the sense of the separate self are completely transcended.

When you enter deeper levels of samadhi, the very essence of the object of meditation is revealed. As it matures into the next stage of *nirvikalpa samadhi*, one enters complete absorption— the individual drop of water merges and becomes one with the vastness of the ocean.

As you progressively enter deeper absorption, the doer disappears. This is when the performer disappears into the performance. The dancer disappears into the dance, thus the sense of self-consciousness is transcended and the powers of the Higher Self flood through the performance. Here the dance is merely the medium for emptying self-concepts and identification with the history or the future of the self. The state of samadhi occurs when the meditator, the technique of meditation and the object of meditation merge into the experience of oneness.

When the doer disappears, you move from becoming to being. As the mind becomes empty of self-seeking in any form, the miracles of the spirit manifest. The final stage is the absolute union of Shiva and Shakti, which is experienced as the orgasmic ecstasy and unity we call Samadhi.

Glossary

Amrita…from Hindu mythology; a nectar of life. In Sanskrit, the prefix a means "not," the root mrita means "dead." Amrita is the drink of immortality. Immortality is the ultimate stage that yogis aspire to. Amrita is the divine elixir that heals all human suffering caused by separative consciousness.

Acceptance…ceasing resistance, absence of reaction to what is present in reality.

Asanas…yoga postures.

Ashtanga…the eight-limbed yoga system as explained in the Yoga Sutras codified by Patanjali around the 2nd century BC.

Atman…Soul, Higher Self, eternal Source.

Avidya…illusion; ignorance of reality.

Avatar…an incarnation of God.

Awareness…represents the meditative perception of reality without personal bias.

Bhagavad Gita…The Song of the Lord; epic tale depicting Krishna's discourse to his beloved disciple, Arjuna, as he prepares to go into battle.

Bhakti Yoga…The yoga of love, devotion and selfless service.

Chakras…The seven centers (wheels) of energy/consciousness located in the subtle body, where we receive, transmit, and process life energies (see prana). The chakras are astral centers, corresponding to the nerve plexuses in the spine. Each chakra has specific characteristics corresponding to a particular state of consciousness.

Choiceless awareness...(See Witness Consciousness.)

Darshan...an audience with a spiritual master or a saint.

Direct experience....experiencing directly without the interference or distortion from preprogrammed personal biases; experience beyond the rational mind with beginner's mind, which is received at a cellular level.

Duality...when natural polarity is altered by personal preferences for or against what is present, it becomes duality. Through this personal preference, the complementary polarity in nature becomes conflicting duality for those who attempt to separate one pole from the other, which is experienced as internal conflict. (See Polarity.)

Dharma...spiritual truth, natural law; the way of truth.

Dharana...concentration, one of the eight limbs of Ashtanga Yoga. Part of the mental discipline of Raja Yoga.

Dhyana...meditation; one of the eight limbs of Ashtanga Yoga. It is the entrance to the spiritual dimension of the discipline of Ashtanga Yoga.

Enlightenment...liberation; absolute freedom; awakening of the Self.

Ecstasy...derived from the Greek, "to stand outside of oneself." In yoga, it is the ultimate orgasmic experience of the union of Shiva and Shakti, known as Samadhi. It is the experience of union with the Self that has been completely liberated from the limitations of the self-image.

Ego...the self-image, which comes to us through the mind and our preprogrammed self-concepts and belief systems.

Experiential...(See Direct experience.)

Hatha Yoga...represents a physical component of the mental and spiritual discipline of Raja Yoga. Together, they form Patanjali's classical system of eight-limbed Ashtanga Yoga.

Integration...the process of bringing together the physical, mental, emotional and spiritual bodies to function and act in complete balance and harmony as a unit. Integration (union) is the basic purpose of the practice of yoga.

Japa...recitation of mantra, often in conjunction with mala (prayer) beads.

Karma...the law of cause and effect: every action has an opposite and equal reaction. "As you sow, so shall you reap." Karma is the experience of unresolved, incomplete experiences of the past, returning again and again in the present, giving us new opportunities to encounter it consciously and resolve it. The action we perform is called karma and the reaction to the action that we experience is the result of karma.

Kriyas...spontaneous physical manifestations directly activated by awakened Kundalini in the form of Hatha Yoga postures, pranayamas, locks, mudras, and cleansing kriyas, leading toward the highest state of samadhi.

Kundalini...the primordial cosmic energy that lies coiled at the base of the spine. When awakened, Kundalini begins to move upward, penetrating the chakras and initiating various yogic kriyas, which bring about total purification, rejuvenation and transformation of the entire being, leading to the ultimate state of samadhi, the state of immortality.

Mantra...powerful sound vibrations which, when chanted continuously, have a calming and purifying effect on the nervous system, mind and heart; sacred sounds of power which release potent spiritual energies within the chanter; a sacred incantation.

Meditation...objective impersonal observation of whatever becomes the object of our awareness; the development of non-judgmental witness which allows us to embrace opposites unconditionally and takes us from the field of duality to the sacred state of unity and oneness.

Meditative Awareness...(See Witness Consciousness.)

Mudras...various hand gestures and physical positions prompted spontaneously by the awakened Kundalini that create internal movement of the energy to mobilize and direct the energies to break through blockages in the physical, mental and emotional bodies.

Nadi Shuddhi...through consistent practice of asanas, pranayama, diet, and a balanced way of living, the body is relaxed, nerve channels are refined, blood is purified, the mind is clear and calm, the heart is open and receptive to subtler vibrations. Its purity radiates through sparkling eyes, clear radiant countenance and luminosity of the skin.

Nirvikalpa Samadhi...complete absorption; the thought-less formless state of being.

Nivritti Marg...yogic path of renunciation.

Om...the primordial sound, which represents unity; the essence of all mantras.

Patanjali...often called the Father of Yoga; first to formally record yogic practices as the eight limbs of yoga, circa 200 BC; his exposition is called the Yoga Sutras.

Polarity...in nature, polarity is complementary and operates in harmony as a unit (one pole cannot exist without the other); it exists in the form of attraction and repulsion, birth and death, expansion and contraction. (See Duality.)

Prana...the primal intelligent energy that regulates the macrocosm of the entire universe as well as the universe in microcosm–the human body; represents the soul as well as the vital breath.

Prana pranotthana...postures are performed automatically when prana has been awakened in the body of a yogi; this is the entrance into Kundalini yoga.

Pranav...chanting of OM with a closed mouth.

Pranayama...breathing techniques that regulate, control and restrain the breath; one of the disciplines of yoga that extend the power of prana.

Pratyahara...retrieving outgoing attention, one of the eight limbs of Ashtanga Yoga.

Pravritti Marg...yogic path of the householder.

Puja...rituals of worship.

Raja Yoga...the mental discipline of yoga.

Rishis...ancient yogis, seers who had a direct experience or perception of God.

Sadhana...all spiritual practices.

Saha...the mundane world; the physical plane.

Samadhi...the eighth limb of Ashtanga Yoga; the final experience of the ultimate union of the individual soul with the cosmic soul.

Satsang...in the company of truth (literal); a devotional gathering.

Savikalpa Samadhi...meditation experience of bliss but with awareness of the object of experience; the beginning stage of samadhi.

Self...soul that denotes both Supreme soul as well as individual soul; according to ancient Vedantic scriptures, both are identical.

Self-Discovery...the process of disassociating from identification with our self-image as our Self; uncovering all the masks and layers to reveal the Self that is hidden behind the self-image.

Sensation (bodily)...ability to feel what is present without the preprogrammed preference for or against the experience; it is a felt-sense experience.

Separative Ego...the self-image, which is born of our self-concepts. When we identify with our self-image as our true self, we are separated from ourselves, from others, and from our Higher Self.

Seva...selfless service; fosters an attitude of selflessness and spiritual awareness.

Shanti...Peace.

Shakti...the female force or energy. It is the divine cosmic energy, which projects, maintains and dissolves the universe; portrayed as the universal mother.

Shiva...consciousness; also a name for the all-pervasive supreme reality; one of the Hindu trinity, representing the process of transformation.

Shushumna...subtle nerve channel within the spinal column, extending from the base of the spine to the brain through which awakened Kundalini rises; it is the pathway to the ultimate experience of yoga–union.

Surrender...letting go of the ego (self); willingness to be open and to wholeheartedly embrace all experiences without judgment. Surrender is letting go of all that holds us back from being one with our divine Self.

Sutra...thread, a line of thought.

Swasthya...ultimate health; being established in the inborn
self-generative, self-healing power of our physical,
mental and emotional bodies.

Tapas...the burning of unconscious activities; adopting the
specific discipline of yoga with the intention to burn
all karma. When it burns it creates heat, irritation, fear,
resistance, self-defense, desire to blame.

Third Eye...the sacred spot between the eyebrows where
integration occurs; its location is the sixth chakra.

Upanishads...summaries of the teachings in the Vedas; the
Amrit Yoga opening prayer is from this scripture.

Vedas...the four ancient scriptures upon which Hinduism is
based; also knowledge, wisdom.

Witness Consciousness...non-participative choiceless
awareness or meditative awareness–the non-judgmental,
impersonal observer.

Yamas and Niyamas...abstentions and guidelines that help
protect us and prevent distractions and disturbances
that come from within and from without.

Yoga...union of the individual soul with the cosmic soul; the
ecstatic experience of the union of Shiva and Shakti; the
state of oneness with the Higher Self.

Yoga Nidra...a conscious connection with your
subconscious where you enter the alpha state; in
this state the mystical powers of the Third Eye are
released, actualizing the healing power of affirmations,
visualizations and prayers.

Zen...the enigmatic state of unity with all that is.

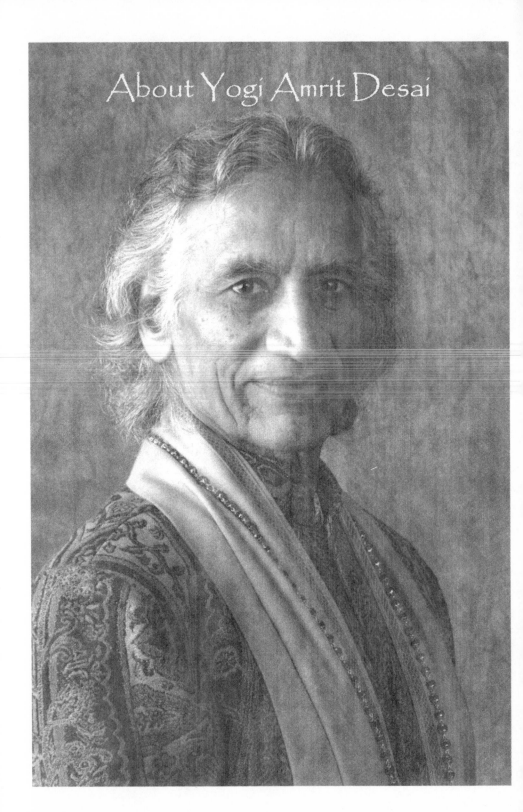

About Yogi Amrit Desai

Yogi Amrit Desai is an internationally renowned yoga master, seminar leader and author in the field of yoga and holistic living. Widely acknowledged for carrying the true and authentic voice of yoga to the world, he has been honored with such rare awards as: "Doctor of Yoga" by H.H. Shankaracharaya, "Jagadacharaya" (Universal Teacher) by the World Religious Parliament in New Delhi, and the "Vishwa Yoga Ratna" awarded by the President of India. He was also nominated for "Padma Vibhushan," the highest honor of India, by former Prime Minister Chandra Shekhar.

Yogi Desai is one of the earliest pioneers of yoga in America. Following his profound life-transforming Kundalini awakening, he developed a methodology that altered the popular notion of yoga as a physical discipline and reintroduced a spiritual dimension to the practice of Hatha Yoga. He named this approach Kripalu Yoga: Meditation in Motion, in honor of his guru.

The yoga society Yogi Desai founded in 1966 eventually grew into the Kripalu Center for Yoga and Health, one of the largest centers of its kind in America. The methodology he developed has become widely adopted and is taught and practiced by thousands around the world.

Yogi Desai continues to develop and teach his innovative approach in the form of Amrit Yoga. What distinguishes Amrit Yoga from Kripalu Yoga is the refinement and distillation of his methodology over the past 30 years. Amrit Yoga has evolved from Kripalu Yoga just as Kripalu Yoga evolved through Yogi Desai's teachings over the years.

The most important aspect of Amrit Yoga is receiving it directly from its creator. There is no greater source of inspiration than learning from a living master.

Redesign Your Destiny...

The Amrit Yoga Institute offers Yoga Alliance-approved yoga teacher certifications in two 10-day courses (200 and 500-hours) and the Amrit Method® Yoga Nidra Professional trainings. All our programs, including the new Zero Stress Zone™ and Quantum Breath Meditations have the potential to deepen personal spiritual development, as well as enhance the skills of yoga teachers from all traditions.

In Amrit Yoga, flexibility of the body is secondary to sourcing the powers of the spirit within. Adding the spiritual dimension to yoga practice takes the practitioners to a whole new level of Self-awareness and Consciousness of the Divine that exists within us all. This is a unique opportunity to learn directly for a world-renowned yoga master—it is an experience that can alter your life forever.

Yogi Desai's CDs, audio and videotapes on guided yoga, meditation, chanting and Yoga Nidra, as well as his lectures on topics about living consciously are available through www.amritkala.com

For more information, contact
The Amrit Yoga Institute
PO Box 5340
Salt Springs, FL   32134
352.685.3001
info@amrityoga.org

Get updated program schedules, new classes and articles on our website: www.amrityoga.org